THE ALCHEMY OF WELLNESS

BRIDGING ANCIENT WISDOM AND MODERN HEALING

ERIKA INDRANI HAWLEY

CONTENTS

DEDICATION

To ALL of my wonderful patients, clients, and students over the years...
THIS ONE IS FOR YOU! I hope you find it fun and helpful.

Thank you for sharing your most tender moments and for allowing me the privilege of being of service all these years.

"May this guide be a steady companion, nurturing your inner wellspring of health and vitality through every season of your life."

To my Dear Family and Husband, Gere
Thank you for showing me a beautiful life and what it truly means to love and be loved. I love you!

PREFACE

In our fast-paced, modern world, it's easy to lose touch with the natural rhythms that sustain us. We often find ourselves out of sync—not just with the cycles of nature, but with our own bodies, minds, spirits, relationships and life purpose.

The truth is, we are part of the same tapestry as the changing seasons, the sun and moon, the shifting tides, and the deep stillness of winter. When we reconnect with this primal rhythm, we rediscover our capacity for balance, joy, and vibrant health.

The Alchemy of Wellness was born from a deep desire to provide a guide back to that connection—to help weave ancient wisdom into modern life and honor the profound interplay between nature, our senses, and our well-being.

This book is my heartfelt offering of that journey to you.

It is not a book of rigid prescriptions or quick fixes. Instead, it is an invitation—an opportunity to slow down, notice, and reawaken to the magic that exists all around and within us.

HOW THIS BOOK IS STRUCTURED

The book is divided into five parts, each offering perspectives, practices, and inspiration to help you align with the rhythms of nature and your own inner wisdom.

Journey through the five elements and the seasonal cycles of life, blending Chinese Medicine, Yoga, Aromatherapy, Sensory Awareness, and Nutrition into a holistic approach to well-being.

It is meant to be read at your own pace, through different lenses-whether you choose to follow the seasons in real-time or dive in to specific chapters or senses that call to you.

I hope it offers a neurodivergent landscape for you to explore within these pages.

AN INVITATION TO EMBARK ON THIS JOURNEY

Let it **be your companion, not a task.**

An invitation to try a practice here and there, savor the process, and listen to how your body and life respond to your participation!

You might also return to certain sections, practices or recipes repeatedly, using them as a guide and reminder when life calls for renewal, grounding, nourishment or introspection.

REAWAKEN YOUR INNER WISDOM

Ultimately, this journey is about remembering what has always been true—you are inherently connected to nature, and your body holds an innate wisdom that modern life often clouds.

While this book is not the only one to explore these practices and principles, my hope is that it offers you a practical and accessible guide to integrating them into your everyday life, through every season.

As you walk this path, may you come to realize what I wholeheartedly believe: *"Wellness" is not about attaining perfection—it is about moving in rhythm with the natural cycles of life.*

May these pages serve as a guide, an inspiration, and a gentle reminder that change, imperfection, and transformation are not obstacles but essential aspects of our beautifully intricate journey.

Let this book nourish and support you as you step into your own unique expression of *The Alchemy of Wellness*—fully embracing the magic of your own wild and precious life.

With love, gratitude, and reverence,

Erika "Indrani" Hawley, L.Ac., MSAOM, RYT

ACKNOWLEDGMENTS

Writing *The Alchemy of Wellness* has been an extraordinary journey of reflection, learning, and connection over these last few years, and it would not have been possible without the support, inspiration, and wisdom of so many incredible people. I extend my deepest gratitude to the following individuals and communities who have shaped, encouraged, and guided me along the way.

To my patients and students- Your stories, dedication, and courage to embrace transformation have been my greatest teachers. Thank you for entrusting me as a guide on your healing journeys and for showing me the infinite wisdom of the human spirit.

To my family and friends- Thank you for your unwavering support, for believing in me, and for giving me the space to create, reflect, and grow through life. I love you all!

To my mentors and teachers- From the masters of Chinese medicine and Yoga philosophy to those who have shared the art of aromatherapy, nutrition, and holistic wellness—your teachings have inspired the foundation of this book and my life. A special thank you to my teachers at the Bihar School of Yoga and connected sangha, whose traditions and presence have deepened my understanding of the interplay between body, mind, and spirit and changed the course of my life for the better.

To my colleagues in the healing arts- Thank you for sharing your knowledge, insights, and passion for holistic health! Your dedication to integrating ancient wisdom with modern science is incredible and inspiring. I hope this book supports your efforts in teaching, keeping yourself in balance, and learning something new or familiar in a new way!

To the ancient traditions and wisdom keepers- My deepest gratitude goes to the lineage of Chinese medicine practitioners, Yogic sages, herbalists, Native Peoples around the world and natural healers who have preserved and shared their wisdom over the centuries. This book is a humble effort to honor the teachings I have received from you and convey the essence of these practices in a simple, transformative way.

To my literary collaborators- my editors, designers, and the publishing team—thank you for helping bring my ideas to life with care, creativity, and precision. Your expertise has been invaluable in shaping this book into formation.

To the natural world- The seasons, the Elementals, and the sensory gifts of life—thank you for being my ultimate teacher and inspiration. Your rhythms and wisdom are woven into every page of this work. And I thank you especially winter, for the necessary moments of stillness to compete this book.

To my ancestors- To the wise and loving spirits of my lineage, Sami, Norwegian, Latvian, English, Finnish and Scottish-thank you for guiding me, protecting me, and inspiring me to remember my connection to you, to my lineage, to the Mother Earth, and the eternal spirals of life.

To my readers- Thank you for choosing to embark on this journey with me! Your curiosity, openness, and commitment to personal growth inspire everything I do. I am deeply grateful to share these teachings with you and to walk alongside you as we explore the beauty and magic of life together. I hope you enjoy the journey!

This book is a reflection of the love, wisdom, and energy of all those who have touched my life.

Blessings and heartfelt thanks to you all!

PART I
THE FOUNDATIONS OF SENSORY ALCHEMY

Our journey begins with Awakening to the Senses and understanding their profound connection to the natural world. The ancient traditions of Chinese Medicine, and Yogic philosophy teach that everything in existence is woven together through the dance of elements, seasons, and energy systems. When we learn to attune ourselves to these rhythms, we begin to experience life in a more balanced and harmonious way.

You'll explore the dynamic interplay of Wood, Fire, Earth, Metal, and Water, the principles of Yin and Yang, and how science and ancient traditions can work together to support balance. As well as guidance for how to create sacred space—a foundation for deep healing and transformation.

1 AWAKENING THE SENSES

"Our senses are not mere conduits for perceiving the world around us; they are powerful gateways to our innermost selves"

-Erika Hawley

Bridging Ancient Knowledge and Seasonal Healing

Throughout history, ancient cultures recognized the deep connection between our senses and our ability to thrive. They understood that our senses are not just individual experiences but are woven into the fabric of our existence—shaping our physical, emotional, and spiritual well-being while influencing how we interact with the world.

In today's fast-paced world, we often disconnect from these natural ways of sensing, healing, and staying balanced. However, by consciously engaging with our senses, we can cultivate a profound awareness of our inner and outer worlds.

This chapter explores the link between our senses and the principles of Traditional Chinese Medicine (TCM), revealing how each sense corresponds to an element, organ system, and season. By understanding these relationships, we can align with nature's rhythms and foster deeper harmony within ourselves.

Have you ever stepped outside on a beautiful day and felt drawn to pause, breathe in the air, or touch the surrounding foliage or earth?

These simple moments of sensory connection are more than just fleeting experiences—they are invitations into presence and healing.

By intentionally engaging with our senses, we enrich our lives, enhance our well-being, and rediscover the innate wisdom that connects us to nature.

THE FIVE SENSES AND THEIR ELEMENTAL CONNECTIONS IN CHINESE MEDICINE

Sense of Sight | Wood Element

Sight is connected to the Wood element, which governs growth, vision, and flexibility. The Liver and Gallbladder meridians regulate detoxification, decision-making, and the smooth flow of Qi (energy). Just as trees stretch toward the sky, our ability to "see" clearly—both physically and metaphorically—depends on a healthy Liver.

Key Organ Functions:

- **Liver:** Ensures smooth Qi flow and stores blood.
- **Gallbladder:** Aids in decision-making and clarity.

Ways to Balance:

- Spend time outdoors, allowing natural light to refresh your vision.
- Eat leafy greens and sour foods to support Liver health.
- Engage in creative activities like journaling or visualization exercises.

Sense of Taste | Fire Element

Taste is governed by the Fire element, which is associated with the Heart and Small Intestine meridians. Fire represents passion, warmth, and transformation—qualities reflected in how flavors bring excitement and nourishment to our bodies.

Key Organ Functions:

- **Heart:** Regulates emotions, circulation, and vitality.
- **Small Intestine:** Sorts and assimilates nutrients, filtering what is beneficial.

Ways to Balance:

- Enjoy warm, vibrant foods like spices, bitter greens, and citrus.
- Engage in heart-opening activities such as singing, laughing, or spending time with loved ones.
- Savor meals mindfully, appreciating their flavors and energy.

Sense of Touch | Earth Element

The sense of touch is deeply linked to the Earth element, which governs nourishment, stability, and connection. In TCM, the Spleen and Stomach meridians play a vital role in digestion, energy absorption, and the body's ability to feel supported. Touch provides grounding and security, much like the Earth provides a foundation for life.

Key Organ Functions:

- **Spleen:** Transforms food into Qi and blood.
- **Stomach:** Processes and distributes nutrients.

Ways to Balance:

- Walk barefoot on natural surfaces like grass or soil.

- Practice grounding techniques like self-massage or acupressure.
- Eat nourishing, whole foods such as root vegetables and grains.

Sense of Smell | Metal Element

Smell is governed by the Metal element, which is linked to the Lungs and Large Intestine meridians. Metal represents refinement, clarity, and the process of release—just as inhalation brings in fresh oxygen and exhalation releases what is no longer needed.

Key Organ Functions:

- **Lungs:** Govern Qi and respiration.
- **Large Intestine:** Eliminates waste and supports detoxification.

Ways to Balance:

- Practice deep breathing exercises, such as diaphragmatic breathing.
- Use essential oils like eucalyptus, frankincense, or peppermint.
- Declutter your environment to encourage a sense of spaciousness.

Sense of Sound | Water Element

The Water element governs the sense of sound and is associated with the Kidneys and Urinary Bladder meridians. Water represents depth, adaptability, and intuition—qualities reflected in how sound waves affect our energy and emotions.

Key Organ Functions:

- **Kidneys:** Store vital essence (Jing) and regulate fluid balance.
- **Urinary Bladder:** Supports elimination and detoxification.

Ways to Balance:

- Listen to calming sounds like ocean waves, rain, or soft music.
- Practice deep breathing and hydration to nourish the Kidney energy.
- Use chanting or vocal toning to promote vibrational healing.

Sense of Intuition | Ether (Spirit) Element

Beyond the five physical senses, the sense of intuition is often linked to the Heart and the Third Eye (Sixth Chakra) in yogic philosophy. In TCM, intuition is associated with Shen (spirit), which resides in the Heart and governs consciousness, wisdom, and higher awareness.

Key Functions:

- **Heart:** Governs emotions and spiritual connection
- **Third Eye:** Enhances perception and intuitive insight.

Ways to Balance:

- Engage in meditation, visualization, or dream journaling.
- Practice mindfulness and deep listening to your inner guidance.
- Trust intuitive feelings and allow space for reflection and self-awareness.

CONCLUSION: HONORING THE WISDOM OF THE SENSES

Chinese medicine teaches us that our senses are more than just ways to perceive the world—they are pathways to balance, healing, and self-discovery. Each sense corresponds to an element, organ system, and natural rhythm, influencing our health on multiple levels.

By aligning our practices with the seasons, we can cultivate greater harmony in body, mind, and spirit. Intentional movement, mindful eating, aromatherapy, breath work, and meditation become tools for seasonal self-care, enhancing our sensory awareness and deepening our connection to nature.

As we move forward, let us embrace our senses as gateways to a richer, more embodied life. By tuning into the wisdom they offer, we rediscover the profound healing available to us—within and all around us.

2

DANCE OF ELEMENTS-WOOD, FIRE, EARTH, METAL, WATER

"The dance is not where we lose ourselves. But where we find ourselves."
-Gabrielle Roth

Our Elemental Allies

In the East and various ancient traditions, the five elements —Wood, Fire, Earth, Metal, and Water—are not only seen as the building blocks of the universe but also as a profound reflection of the natural world and human experience within us. These elements are intricately intertwined with the ever-changing seasons and our bodies, creating a dynamic interplay between nature and our own internal landscapes. I like to think of them simply as elemental "friends".

Understanding the connection between the elements and seasons and our sensory experience can provide us with valuable insights into maintaining balance and cultivating health throughout the year.

THE SPIRAL OF LIFE AND THE ELEMENTS: A JOURNEY OF TRANSFORMATION

The spiral is one of the most ancient and sacred symbols found across cultures, representing the continuous cycle of growth, transformation, and evolution. In the context of the Five Elements of Chinese Medicine—Wood, Fire, Earth, Metal, and Water—the spiral beautifully illustrates how these forces interact, shift, and flow into one another in a rhythmic, never-ending dance. Just as nature follows spiraling patterns—from the unfurling of a fern to the galaxies in the cosmos—our own healing, transformation, and personal evolution move in spirals rather than in straight lines.

I have always been fascinated by the spirals in a persons fingerprints and in nature in so many forms. My maiden name is Eddy and I used to find that funny to contemplate how being an "eddy" expressed in my own nature through this lense lol. An "Eddie" in slang terms is "a whirlpool against the direction of the current"- a feeling I have often had through my life ironically! And one that has taught me a lot about going *with* the flow of life.

SACRED GEOMETRY AND THE SPIRAL: THE BLUEPRINT OF NATURE

Sacred geometry is the mathematical language of the universe, revealing the fundamental patterns that underlie all of creation. Among the most significant geometric forms is the spiral, which appears in the Fibonacci sequence, the golden ratio (Phi), and the swirling galaxies above and ocean shells below. These forms are not just beautiful; they are blueprints of the life force that governs energy, movement, and transformation.

The spiral is both a symbol and a process—one that mirrors the generating cycle of the Five Elements in Chinese Medicine and our own personal and spiritual evolution.

The Fibonacci Spiral in Nature: This spiral pattern follows a precise mathematical sequence, where each number is the sum of the two preceding ones (0, 1, 1, 2, 3, 5, 8, 13, 21, 34...). This sequence is found in everything from the arrangement of sunflower seeds to the branching of trees and the proportions of the human body.

The Golden Ratio and Balance: The Golden Ratio (1.618) is considered a divine proportion, reflecting harmony, balance, and beauty in everything from ancient architecture to the symmetry of the human face. In healing practices like Chinese Medicine, Yoga, and Ayurveda, balance is the key to vitality and longevity.

The Spiral in the Human Energy Field: The body's energy centers, or chakras, also move in a spiraling vortex of energy, pulling in and radiating out life force (Qi or Prana). The Torodial Field ("Torus") surrounding the heart and the body operates on these same sacred geometric principles, reminding us that energy is not static but in constant movement and flux.

The Spiral as a Journey of Transformation: Just as sacred geometry reflects the perfection and intelligence of the natural world, the spiral reminds us that our path is not linear. True transformation happens in cycles, as we spiral through the seasons of life, learning, unlearning, and evolving with greater wisdom at each turn.

THE SPIRAL AS A PATH OF GROWTH AND CHANGE

Unlike linear progress, which suggests a direct and final destination, the spiral reminds us that life is a continuous process of learning, shedding, and renewal. Each turn of the spiral brings us back to similar themes or lessons—but from a higher or deeper perspective, offering us new insight and awareness.

Through the seasons and elements, we witness the eternal flow of energy:

Spring (Wood Element) – Expansion and Ascent: Just like the spiral's outward movement, Wood represents new growth, rising energy, and forward movement. It is the phase of rebirth and vision, much like a sprouting seed reaching for the sky.

Summer (Fire Element) – Radiance and Full Expression: As the spiral expands outward, Fire represents the height of energy, passion, and connection. It is the time of full bloom, joy, and dynamic transformation, much like the peak of the spiral's movement outward into the world.

Late Summer (Earth Element) – Integration and Centering: At the center of the spiral is Earth, the grounding force that reminds us to pause, assimilate, and nourish ourselves. This phase stabilizes the transition between expansion (Fire) and contraction (Metal), ensuring that we are supported and centered before the next shift.

Autumn (Metal Element) – Refinement and Release: Just as a spiral turns inward, Metal draws energy back to its core, symbolizing discernment, clarity, and letting go. Like leaves falling from trees, this phase reminds us that releasing is necessary for renewal.

Winter (Water Element) – Stillness and Deep Reflection: The spiral turns even deeper inward as Water represents a return to the source, introspection, and conservation of energy. This is the phase of inner alchemy, where wisdom is gathered before the next cycle of rebirth.

THE SPIRAL AND OUR PERSONAL EVOLUTION

We do not move through the elements and seasons in rigid steps but rather in a flowing, spiraling journey. We may revisit the same lessons, emotions, or challenges at different points in life, yet each time we arrive, we do so with new perspectives, greater resilience, and deeper wisdom.

This spiral path invites us to trust the process—to embrace both expansion and contraction, knowing that each phase serves its purpose. It teaches us to honor both movement and stillness, action and surrender, growth and rest.

By aligning with the spiraling rhythm of nature, we begin to see that healing, transformation, and self-discovery are not about reaching an endpoint—they are about learning to move with the rhythm of life, embracing the ever-changing, spiraling dance of existence. The spiral is present at each energy point along our acupuncture meridians and our Chakras- wheels or vorteces of energy that are constantly interacting.

THE GENERATING CYCLE: THE ALCHEMY OF TRANSFORMATION IN CHINESE MEDICINE

In Traditional Chinese Medicine (TCM), the Generating Cycle, also known as the Sheng Cycle, illustrates the continuous transformation and interdependence of the Five Elements—Wood, Fire, Earth, Metal, and Water. This cycle represents the natural rhythm of life, where each element nurtures and gives rise to the next, ensuring harmony in both nature and the human body.

- **Wood generates Fire** as trees provide fuel for flames to burn.
- **Fire generates Earth** as ashes decompose and enrich the soil.
- **Earth generates Metal** as minerals and ores form within its depths.
- **Metal generates Water** as minerals condense and direct the flow of water.
- **Water generates Wood** as moisture nourishes seeds and enables plants to grow.

This continuous process reflects the profound wisdom of nature—where destruction gives way to renewal, and each phase supports the next in an endless cycle of creation. Within our bodies, this cycle governs the relationships between organ systems, emotions, and energetic pathways. When it flows smoothly, we experience vitality, emotional balance, and resilience. However, if disrupted, stagnation, deficiency, or imbalance may arise.

By aligning our lifestyle, diet, and movement practices with the natural rhythm of the elements, we can cultivate greater harmony within ourselves and the world around us.

The Generating Cycle serves as a reminder that transformation is an essential part of life's alchemy—guiding us toward growth, renewal, and the wisdom of change.

THE DANCE OF ELEMENTS: ALIGNING WITH NATURE'S RHYTHMS

Our senses—sight, sound, smell, taste, and touch—are windows into the richness of the world around us. By tuning into them, we can deepen our awareness and experience the beauty, depth, and vitality of life. This book invites you to explore how each season mirrors the natural elements in Traditional Chinese Medicine and how aligning with these rhythms can bring balance to your body, mind, and spirit.

In spring, the Wood element awakens, embodying growth, renewal, and expansion. Just as trees send out new shoots, our energy rises, sparking creativity and action. Spring invites us to focus on SIGHT, vision, planning, and movement—Nature's true New Year. Embodiment practices that stimulate the Wood element, such as side bends, abdominal twists, and joint-opening poses, support flexibility and detoxification. Deep, invigorating breaths and time spent in nature help us embrace the upward-rising energy of this season.

As we transition into summer, the Fire element ignites, bringing joy, vitality, and connection. This season encourages us to celebrate, express ourselves, and cultivate relationships. Expansive, heart-opening poses like backbends, flowing movements, and gentle dancing align with Fire's energy, while gratitude meditations nourish the heart and promote balance. Moments of pause and reflection are key to tempering Fire's intensity and fostering a sense of inner warmth without burnout.

Late summer bridges the transition between summer and autumn, embodying the Earth element—stability, nourishment, and balance.

It is a time for grounding, centering, and deep self-care. Practices that emphasize standing balance poses, restorative forward bends, and longer-held stretches help cultivate steadiness. Breathing techniques like Alternate Nostril Breathing or the 4:7:8 breath ratio bring calmness, particularly if the lingering heat of summer feels overstimulating.

As autumn arrives, the Metal element invites refinement and release. Like leaves falling from the trees, this season encourages us to let go of what no longer serves us and cultivate clarity. Breath-centered practices, meditation, and introspection align with Metal's energy. Chest-opening poses and gentle twists help clear the lungs and intestines, supporting both physical and emotional release. This is a time to create space for what is essential.

Finally, winter embodies the Water element, a season of rest, introspection, and energy conservation. Just as nature slows down, winter invites us to turn inward, reflect, and replenish. Gentle, warming yoga poses and restorative practices nurture the Water element, while meditation and stillness help us connect with deep inner wisdom. By honoring the quiet energy of winter, we prepare for the renewal that follows in spring.

By recognizing and embracing this cyclical dance of the elements, we attune ourselves to nature's rhythms, finding harmony, resilience, and a deeper connection to life itself. Through intentional movement, breath work, and sensory awareness, we align with the changing seasons, cultivating well-being in a way that is both grounding and expansive. When we move in sync with nature, we rediscover the flow of life within and around us, allowing each season to guide us toward balance, renewal, and growth.

3
SEASONAL CONNECTION TO HEALTH

"All the trees are losing their leaves, and not one of them is worried."
- Donald Miller

Acknowledging our connection to Nature

Human beings have always been intrinsically linked to the natural world, a connection that is both intuitive and necessary. While many of us may still feel this connection, modern societies with their concrete landscapes and bustling urban environments, have distanced many from the natural elements that sustain us. The vast expanses of concrete and sky have, for a large majority of humans, replaced the more intimate relationship with the earth that our ancestors once had. And unlike the above quote, the modern person tends to get very worried about changes and the act of "letting go".

Yet, despite this physical separation, nature continues to be the framework—the fabric—upon which we live and thrive.

As modern humans, we have become disconnected from the rhythms and wisdom of nature, which, in turn, affects our sense of wholeness and well-being. Nature is not just the backdrop of our lives but the very weft and warp that weave together the human experience. The interconnectedness of the mind, body, and spirit mirrors the interdependent systems of nature, where every element is aligned with the cycles of life. These seasonal rhythms not only govern the world around us but also influence the flow of energy within us.

Eastern philosophies, particularly those embedded in Traditional Chinese Medicine (TCM) and ancient Yogic traditions, emphasize that the body is a microcosm of the universe. These ancient perspectives observe the seasons and natural phenomena as key to understanding our own inner workings. The body, mind, and spirit are interconnected in a dance with the natural world—when we align with the flow of life, we achieve balance, health, and harmony.

By attuning ourselves to these natural rhythms, we can restore alignment and feel more integrated within our environment. Just as nature evolves and adapts, so must we. When we adopt simple tools and practices to cultivate resilience, vitality, and a deep sense of connection, we begin to thrive—even in the face of life's inevitable shifts and changes. The essence of living a balanced life lies in understanding and honoring the cycles of nature, especially the seasons.

CYCLES OF THE SEASONS: A FRAMEWORK FOR GROWTH AND HEALING

The seasons reflect the cyclical nature of existence. Each season brings with it a unique energy, perspective, and opportunity for growth. Just like the turning of the year, our lives also go through cycles—moments of growth, expansion, contraction, and rest. Seasons serve as a natural framework for the chapters of our lives, offering us the chance to attune our activities, habits, and mindset to the ever-changing energy of nature. When we align with these shifts, we can harness their inherent wisdom and receive the gifts they bring with ease and flow.

SPRING: RENEWAL AND GROWTH

Spring represents new beginnings, rebirth, and expansion. It is a time for planting the seeds of our dreams, ideas, and goals and nurturing them into the future. Spring embodies the Wood element in Chinese medicine, symbolizing growth, vitality, and the flourishing of new life. The natural world is awakening—buds bloom, animals come out from hibernation, and the air is filled with new possibilities.

When in Balance: In spring, ideally you feel energized, optimistic, and open to new experiences. Your body feels refreshed, and there's a sense of new potential in your life.

**If you're not feeling these qualities—if you're still holding onto old habits, emotional baggage, or stuck energy—it may indicate a blockage that needs addressing.

Signs of Imbalance:

- **Physical Symptoms:** Muscle stiffness, headaches, eye strain, allergies, sluggish digestion, or liver congestion.
- **Emotional Symptoms:** Irritability, frustration, impatience, or feeling easily overwhelmed.
- **Mental Symptoms:** Indecisiveness, lack of motivation, creative blockages, or feeling stuck in old habits.
- **Spiritual Symptoms:** Resistance to change, difficulty letting go of past grievances, or struggling to set new intentions.

Tips for Realignment:

Support the Wood element by moving your body, practicing deep breathing, and engaging in creative outlets. Detoxify both physically (light, cleansing foods) and emotionally (letting go of limiting beliefs). Embrace adaptability and new perspectives.

SUMMER: JOY, EXPANSION, AND VITALITY

Summer brings warmth, abundance, and joy. It's the time of full expression, when energy is at its peak, and the world around us seems to burst with vibrancy. The Fire element, associated with the Heart and Small Intestine, governs summer, and it is a time for play, creativity, and social connection.

When in Balance: During summer, you feel expansive, joyful, and full of life. Your creativity flows, and ideally you experience a deep connection with others. You have the energy to spare and feel deeply alive.

**If you're feeling burnt out, exhausted, or disconnected, you may not be fully aligned with the energy of the season, showing the area or element that you need to tend to more.

Signs of Imbalance:

- **Physical Symptoms:** Overheating, inflammation, insomnia, heart palpitations, excessive sweating, or digestive disturbances.
- **Emotional Symptoms:** Anxiety, restlessness, over-excitement, or emotional burnout.
- **Mental Symptoms:** Difficulty focusing, scattered thoughts, or being overly driven without enough rest.
- **Spiritual Symptoms:** Feeling disconnected from joy, lacking meaningful social connections, or struggling with self-expression.

Tips for Realignment:

Balance excess heat with cooling foods and calming activities. Avoid overexertion and make time for relaxation. Focus on heart-centered activities like laughter, gratitude, and connecting with loved ones. Ground your energy with mindful breathing, meditation, and restorative movement.

LATE SUMMER: NOURISHMENT, STABILITY, AND TRANSITION

Late summer is a season of abundance, nourishment, and grounding. It represents a brief but essential pause between the high energy of summer and the cooling, contracting energy of autumn. Governed by the Earth element, this season is associated with the Spleen and Stomach meridians, which are responsible for digestion, assimilation, and a sense of stability—both physically and emotionally. Late summer invites us to center ourselves, gather strength, and integrate the experiences of the past months before moving into the slower, introspective rhythms of fall.

When in Balance:

During late summer, you feel grounded, nourished, and emotionally steady. There is a sense of inner harmony and connection, and you're able to give and receive support with ease. You feel present in your body and able to digest not just food, but also experiences and emotions. Your thoughts are clear, your energy is stable, and your body feels strong and well-nourished.

Signs of Imbalance:

- **Physical Symptoms:** Digestive issues (bloating, nausea, sluggish digestion), sugar cravings, weakened immunity, excessive dampness (phlegm, mucus, water retention), or fatigue.
- **Emotional Symptoms:** Worry, overthinking, feeling overwhelmed, or feeling ungrounded.
- **Mental Symptoms:** Difficulty concentrating, over analyzing, or struggling with decision-making.
- **Spiritual Symptoms:** Lack of connection to self-care, difficulty finding balance between giving and receiving, or feeling energetically depleted.

Tips for Realignment:

Support the Earth element by grounding yourself with nourishing, seasonal foods like root vegetables and warm grains. Reduce excessive worry by practicing mindfulness and engaging in activities that bring a sense of stability, such as yoga, walking in nature, or meditation. Prioritize self-care and ensure you are giving as much as you receive.

AUTUMN: REFLECTION, LETTING GO, AND HARVESTING

As summer wanes, autumn arrives with a sense of transition and introspection. This is the time to let go of what no longer serves us, both physically and emotionally. The Metal element governs autumn, focusing on elimination, boundaries, and reflection. As the leaves fall from the trees, it reminds us to release attachments and make space for the new.

When in Balance: You feel a sense of closure, clarity, and gratitude for what has passed. You are able to reflect on the year, harvest your accomplishments, and prepare for the quieter, inward months ahead. **If you are resisting change or struggling to let go, you may feel stuck, or your energy might feel weighed down in grief or depression.

Signs of Imbalance:

- **Physical Symptoms:** Respiratory issues (coughs, colds, sinus congestion), dry skin, constipation, stiff joints, or weakened immunity.
- **Emotional Symptoms:** Sadness, grief, difficulty letting go, isolation, or feeling disconnected.
- **Mental Symptoms:** Rigid thinking, perfectionism, feeling uninspired, or an inability to move forward.
- **Spiritual Symptoms:** Loss of purpose, struggling with transitions, or difficulty creating space for stillness and reflection.

Tips for Realignment:

Support the Metal element by practicing deep breathing (pranayama), releasing old emotions, and engaging in rituals that help you process grief or transition. Keep warm and hydrated, nourish the lungs with moistening foods, and create space for decluttering—both physically and emotionally.

WINTER: STILLNESS, REST, AND REFLECTION

Winter is the season of rest, reflection, and introspection. It embodies the Water element, symbolizing stillness, rejuvenation, and the deep, quiet wisdom that comes with the cold. In nature, winter is a time for hibernation, for everything to slow down and replenish its energy for the coming year. For us as humans, it is the same- ideally a time to honor the need for slowing down, deep rest and reflection.

When in Balance: You feel calm, centered, and ready for renewal. Your body is at rest, your energy is deepening, and you are in touch with your inner wisdom.

**If you are feeling depressed, lethargic, or restless, it may be a sign that you are resisting the stillness that the winter months offer, or need to shift something to support yourself better.

Signs of Imbalance:

- **Physical Symptoms:** Fatigue, cold extremities, lower back or knee pain, weakened kidney function, sleep disturbances, or water retention.
- **Emotional Symptoms:** Fear, anxiety, insecurity, feeling withdrawn, or lacking trust in life.
- **Mental Symptoms:** Lack of motivation, brain fog, feeling uninspired, or experiencing a sense of stagnation.
- **Spiritual Symptoms:** Disconnection from intuition, resistance to stillness, or feeling lost

Tips for Realignment:

Support the Water element by embracing rest, deep nourishment, and introspection. Prioritize warmth, hydration, and gentle movement like Yin yoga or Qigong. Spend time in meditation, journaling, or other reflective practices. Trust in the natural cycles of life, knowing that winter's stillness is essential for renewal in the coming seasons.

UNDERSTANDING SEASONAL SHIFTS AND THEIR IMPACT ON OUR WELL-BEING

The seasonal changes are more than just the shift of weather or the changing colors of the leaves. They represent powerful, cyclical energy flows that are deeply connected to our own internal rhythms. When we align with the natural world—honoring the energy of each season and adjusting our habits, mindset, and lifestyle accordingly—we create space for greater well-being and fulfillment.

However, when we resist the natural flow of these shifts, it can lead to feelings of disconnection, imbalances, and physical or emotional discomfort. This is why issues like Seasonal Affective Disorder (SAD), burnout, and the "winter blues" occur—when we are out of sync with the energy of the season, or not nourished in some way, we may struggle to feel vibrant and alive.

ALIGNING WITH NATURE'S RHYTHMS: A PATH TO VIBRANT HEALTH

By aligning our lives with the seasonal cycles, we honor our deep connection to nature and ourselves. Understanding the shifts that come with each season and adapting our daily habits, mindsets, and routines accordingly, we become more resilient, balanced, and attuned to our inner wisdom. This practice is not about rigidly following rules but about honoring the flow of life and adapting with grace and ease within your own means and lifestyle goals.

The simple practices, tools, and ideas shared in this book are designed to help you deepen your gratitude and reverence for both your own growth and times of change, as well as the ever-changing beauty of nature.

When we live with an awareness of these natural cycles, we weave ourselves back into the fabric of life, integrating both the wisdom of the seasons and the natural world. In doing so, we remember how to live as a whole, flourishing and thriving, even as the seasons shift around us.

Embrace the cycles of nature, and let them guide you on your journey to wellness, vitality, and harmony. The seasons are not only an external reality; they are a reflection of the rhythm of our inner lives, offering wisdom, healing, and opportunities for growth at every stage.

4

YIN AND YANG- BALANCE OF OPPOSING FORCES

"The principle of Yin and Yang is the foundation of the entire universe. It underlies everything in creation. It brings about the development of parenthood; it is the root and source of life and death; it is found within the temples of the gods. In order to treat and cure diseases one must search for their origins."

- The Yellow Emperors Classic
(Huang Di Nei Jing)

Understanding the Duality of Life

At the heart of Chinese Medicine lies the concept of Yin and Yang, one of the most fundamental and profound theories that explain the interconnectedness and balance of forces within the universe, nature, and the human body. This theory embodies the eternal interplay of opposites, where everything in existence is composed of two opposing yet complementary forces. It is a concept that stretches beyond the boundaries of physical reality into the metaphysical, forming the foundation of not just Chinese Medicine but also of many ancient philosophical and spiritual practices, including Ayurveda and Polarity Therapy.

Much like the force of gravity or the air we breathe—an invisible, ever-present phenomenon governs the movement of objects in the universe.

Yin and Yang govern the natural balance of forces within and around us. These forces are in constant motion and interaction, creating a dynamic tension that drives change, growth, and evolution. Yin and Yang are not static entities but rather dynamic, fluid, and ever-changing aspects of reality.

They are interdependent—one cannot exist without the other. In essence, everything contains the seed of its opposite, and balance between these forces is essential for harmony and health.

YIN AND YANG IN THE HUMAN BODY

In the context of the human body, Yin and Yang represent two sides of the same coin. Yin is associated with qualities such as darkness, stillness, and femininity, while Yang is associated with light, movement, and masculinity. These are not meant to signify good or bad but rather reflect the natural duality in all things. Think of Yin as the night, coolness, or the interior of a cave, and Yang as the day, warmth, or the outward expression of energy. These can also be thought of as being on a spectrum of how much Yin or Yang is present at any given stage.

Each organ system in Traditional Chinese Medicine (TCM) is associated with either Yin or Yang qualities, and together, they work to maintain balance and harmony within the body. This balancing act is essential for the body's health, energy flow, and overall well-being. For example, the Heart is primarily a Yin organ, responsible for circulation, warmth, and expression of energy, while the Small Intestine is a yang organ, representing the activity, breakdown, and movement of toxins and nutrients in the body.

YIN AND YANG IN DAILY LIFE

Every aspect of our daily experience is shaped by Yin and Yang forces, often without us even realizing it. From the rhythms of sleep and wakefulness, activity and rest, to the food we consume, the climate, and the relationships we experience, Yin and Yang play their part in guiding us to balance.

- **Light / Dark:** Our sleep cycle is governed by the Yin and Yang of night and day. We are most active during the day (noon is utmost Yang), and we rest and rejuvenate at night (Midnight is utmost Yin).
- **Heat / Cold:** During the hot summer months (Yang), we feel energized, active, and outward-facing, while in the cold winter (Yin), we seek warmth, quiet, and introspection.
- **Inner / Outer:** We spend a lot of time in the outer world (Yang), expressing our ideas, moving, and interacting with people, but we also need quiet time in the inner world (Yin) for reflection, introspection, and rest.

Yin and Yang don't just oppose one another; they complement and balance each other, offering a way to view how the different aspects of life contribute to our health and stability.

YIN AND YANG IN HEALING AND MEDICINE

In Chinese medicine, balance is key. As it says in the Huang Di Nei Jing, one of the original classics of Chinese Medicine (2500 years old or so), in a conversation with the Yellow Emperor "Huang Di":

"Their first discussion began with Huang Di inquiring, "I've heard that in the days of old everyone lived one hundred years without showing the usual signs of aging. In our time, however, people age prematurely, living only fifty years. Is this due to a change in the environment, or is it because people have lost the correct way of life?"

— **Maoshing Ni,** *The Yellow Emperor's Classic of Medicine: A New Translation of the Neijing Suwen with Commentary*

This quote asks the important question of how our "way of life" may impact health and longevity, or is it our environment, or both? Areas considered "blue zones" in our present day world, offer a great example of this and seem to offer the best balance for living a lifestyle that fosters longevity. I personally believe and have found that environment + lifestyle is key in all cases of achieving modern day longevity and health.

With Yin and Yang, the presence of one force may signal the deficiency or excess of the other, which may lead to imbalance and disease.

When Yang becomes too excessive, it may lead to inflammation, heat, or restlessness. On the other hand, an excess of Yin could lead to coldness, stagnation, or a sense of being depleted. At their extremes, heat turns to cold and cold into heat. To restore health, Chinese Medicine aims to balance both the Yin and Yang within the body.

For example, acupuncture and herbal remedies are used to either strengthen Yin when there is a deficiency or calm excess Yang. Similarly, in Acupuncture or Qigong, we might be aiming to increase or decrease Yang Qi and drain excess or tonify yin.

THE MERIDIAN SYSTEM: THE PATHWAYS OF LIFE FORCE ENERGY (QI)

The meridian system is another essential component in understanding Yin and Yang.

You might think of the meridian system as an energy highway, transporting the vital life force known as Qi (pronounced "chee") throughout the body. The Qi circulates along these pathways, nourishing the organs, tissues, and cells, enabling the body to function at its optimal level.

In Chinese Medicine, the meridian system is closely linked with and affected by the balance of Yin and Yang forces and the elemental cycle of wood, fire, earth, metal and water.

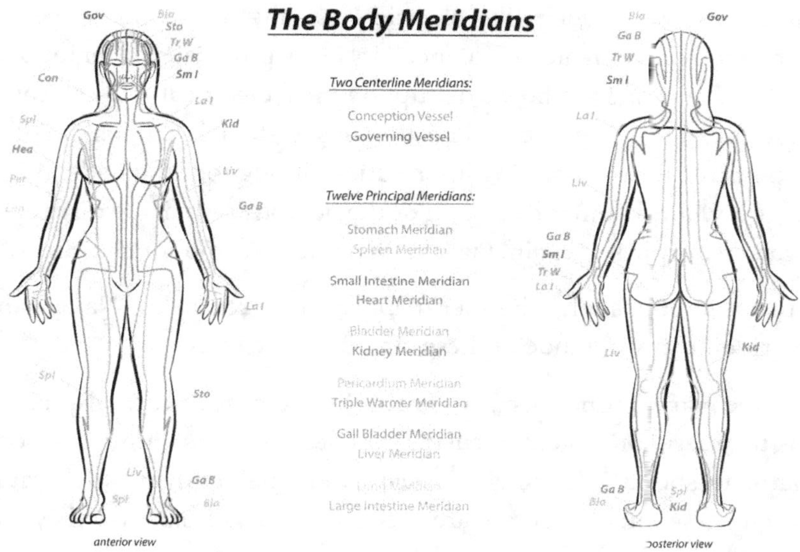

Poster by: PeterHermesFurian

MERIDIANS AND ENERGY FLOW

The body is interwoven with 14 primary meridians, each connected to a specific organ system. These energy channels govern the flow of Qi, ensuring that energy moves smoothly and without obstruction. When Qi flows freely, harmony exists, and the body is in a state of health. However, when there are blockages or imbalances in the meridian system, energy can stagnate, leading to physical or emotional disturbances. This is where practices like acupuncture, Qi Gong, and Yoga come in to restore balance by facilitating the smooth flow of Qi along the meridians.

Each meridian is associated with either a Yin or Yang organ, which influences the flow of Qi and the balance of energy.

For example, the Kidney meridian is more Yin, and it governs vitality, water metabolism, and growth, while its counterpart Urinary Bladder is more Yang, and it governs the release of fluids and movement in the back body.

Meridians work much like electrical circuits, where blockages or disruptions can create imbalances in both physical and emotional health. This is akin to how a disruption in an electrical grid can cause widespread consequences. The nervous system is similar, as it is responsible for transmitting information throughout the body. When the meridian system is disrupted or the nervous system are disrupted, it can create physical pain, tension, dis-ease and emotional distress.

**In Yogic philosophy the meridians are referred to as "Nadis" and they identify over 10,000 of these circuits in the body.

**The chakra (pronounced "CHa-Kra") system from yoga also parallels the meridian system, focusing on energy centers within the body that correspond to various physical, emotional, and spiritual states. When these energy centers are blocked or out of balance, they can manifest as emotional or physical symptoms.

EXERCISE FOR EMBODIMENT: CONNECTING WITH YOUR BODY'S ENERGY FIELD

To better understand the impact of the meridian system and energy flow, try the following exercise to help connect you with the energy pathways running through your body:

1. **Feel your body:** Close your eyes, take a few deep breaths, and bring your awareness to your body.
2. **Notice opposing sensations:** Start by focusing on the right side of your body, then the left side. Feel the differences between the front and back, the head and the feet. Tune in to any tension, warmth, or discomfort.
3. **Pause and observe:** After a few moments, observe the sensations. *Are there areas of imbalance or discomfort? Are*

certain parts of your body more energized than others? What is your experience of opposites or the Yin and Yang right now?

4. **Visualize energy flow:** Imagine your body as a vast network of small river-like channels carrying energy, nutrients, and emotion. From your head to your toes, visualize these channels flowing smoothly. Notice any blockages or stagnant energy that may arise.
5. **Reflection:** After the exercise, take a mental note of how you feel. Do the sensations shift or change as you focus on the flow of Qi? Is there a sense of ease or tension? The more you practice tuning into your body's energy flow, the more connected you become to the underlying currents that sustain your health.

BALANCING THE MERIDIAN SYSTEM TO ENHANCE YOUR HEALING POTENTIAL

By incorporating practices that influence the meridian system, such as acupuncture, yoga, Qi Gong, or Tai Chi, we can enhance the body's natural healing abilities and promote a balanced flow of energy. These practices clear blockages, strengthen weak areas, and restore harmony within the body's energetic network. In doing so, they create a greater sense of well-being, resilience, and vitality, fostering a deeper connection with the vital life force (Qi/Prana) that sustains us.

Moreover, the key to integrating Yin and Yang in your life involves being mindful of balance—balancing rest and activity, stillness and movement, cold and warmth, and outer and inner worlds. When we respect and honor the natural flow of Qi and the inherent duality of Yin and Yang, we can create greater harmony and experience profound healing, both in the body and in our lives.

"The pure Yang forms the heaven, and the turbid Yin forms the earth. The Qi of the earth ascends and turns into clouds, while the Qi of the heaven turns into rain."

— **Maoshing Ni,** *The Yellow Emperor's Classic of Medicine: A New Translation of the Neijing Suwen with Commentary*

CONCLUSION

By understanding and working with the meridian system, Yin and Yang, and Qi, we can enhance our health, develop resilience, and improve our overall life experience. Each of us has the potential to harmonize with the energy of the universe, cultivating vitality and well-being at every level—physical, mental, emotional, and spiritual.

5
INTEGRATING SCIENCE WITH ANCIENT WISDOM

"Future medicine will be the medicine of frequencies."
- Albert Einstein

Bridging Ancient Wisdom and Modern Science

As our understanding of the human brain continues to evolve, the profound connections between ancient wisdom and modern neuroscience become increasingly clear. Neuroscience has begun to shed light on the intricate workings of our neural networks (brain and nervous system), offering deeper insights into how time-honored practices such as Chinese medicine, Yoga, and Aromatherapy influence our well-being.

These practices, which have been revered for millennia, now find scientific validation in the ways they shape and enhance our brain's structure, function, and resilience by quite literally shifting our frequency back into harmony.

The integration of ancient wisdom with the discoveries of modern brain science allows us to better understand the intricate relationships between the mind, body, and spirit. This fusion of knowledge provides an expansive framework for exploring the holistic nature of health and healing. Practices rooted in Chinese medicine, yoga, mindfulness, and the power of the senses not only support physical health but also foster mental clarity and emotional balance.

As we delve deeper into the neuro-scientific foundations of practices that have been passed down for generations, we gain a profound appreciation for their ability to positively influence our biology and the wisdom held by our ancestors.

The convergence of these two worlds—ancient traditions and cutting-edge science—create a powerful synergy for transformation and healing, offering transformative tools for cultivating holistic health.

In this age of rapid scientific progress, the synthesis of ancient knowledge and modern discoveries serve as a beacon for individual and collective well-being.

By understanding the biological mechanisms behind practices like mindfulness, embodiment, and sensory engagement, we gain insights into how to optimize our health and vitality, and unlock the full potential of our mind-body connection.

THE ALCHEMY OF TRANSFORMATION: MERGING ANCIENT WISDOM WITH MODERN HEALING

Alchemy, at its core, is the art of transformation—the process of refining, evolving, and transmuting energy from one state to another. Traditionally, alchemists sought to turn base metals into gold, but beyond the literal interpretation, alchemy represents the profound inner journey of growth, healing, and self-realization. In the context of wellness, alchemy is the practice of blending ancient wisdom, natural cycles, and modern healing modalities to create balance, vitality, and harmony within the body, mind, and spirit.

Just as nature transitions seamlessly through the seasons, we, too, undergo shifts and transformations throughout our lives. By attuning to the elements, honoring the wisdom of Chinese Medicine, Yoga, and Sensory Awareness, and embracing intentional practices such as breath work, movement, meditation, and ritual, we engage in a personal alchemical process—one that transmutes stress into ease, imbalance into wholeness, and disconnection into deep awareness. This is the true essence of The Alchemy of Wellness—a journey of aligning with our innate rhythms, discovering our inner light, and cultivating a life of purpose, harmony, and joy.

In this chapter will explore the alchemical process of healing, how transformation occurs through awareness, integration, and embodiment, and how we can consciously engage with this process to create meaningful, lasting change in our lives.

THE FUTURE OF MEDICINE: THE MEDICINE OF FREQUENCIES

As science and ancient wisdom continue to merge, a growing understanding of vibrational medicine is emerging—one that aligns with the concept that the future of healing will be based on frequency and energy.

Renowned scientist Albert Einstein once said, *"Future medicine will be the medicine of frequencies."* This idea suggests that illness and imbalance are not merely biochemical or physical conditions but also disruptions in the body's energetic field.

In Traditional Chinese Medicine (TCM), Ayurveda, and various indigenous healing systems, the human body is understood as an intricate energy network, where Qi (life force), Prana, and vibrational resonance determine health and well-being.

Modern research is now validating what these traditions have long known—everything in existence carries a specific frequency, including our organs, emotions, thoughts and everything in our physical world.

Healing modalities such as sound therapy, Reiki, Medical Qigong, and bioresonance technology work on the principle that frequencies can be entrained and restored to bring the body back into harmony. Techniques like binaural beats, solfeggio frequencies, tuning forks, and electromagnetic field therapy are being used by individuals to address imbalances at a deep energetic level. Studies suggest that specific sound frequencies can reduce stress, improve brain function, and even aid in tissue regeneration.

The implications of frequency-based medicine are vast, offering a non-invasive, holistic approach to healing. As research continues, we may see a shift from symptom-based treatment to a vibrational model of health, where tuning the body's frequencies—whether through sound, light, bioelectricity, or energy medicine—become the foundation of future medical care.

THE HEART MATH INSTITUTE: WE ARE FREQUENCY-BASED BEINGS

The research conducted by the Heart Math Institute is a compelling example of how modern science and ancient knowledge intersect. Their studies reveal the profound connection between the human nervous system and external geomagnetic activity. Through continuous monitoring of heart rate variability (HRV) and geomagnetic fluctuations, HeartMath found that the autonomic nervous system responds to changes in the solar and geomagnetic fields, suggesting that our bodies are finely tuned to environmental rhythms.

This research highlights how *frequency* plays a central role in regulating our nervous system and overall health. The human body, like the earth, functions on a frequency-based system that is influenced by both internal and external factors. Practices that regulate our internal frequency—such as mindfulness, yoga, and meditation—allow us to synchronize our body's rhythms with those of nature, creating a sense of harmony and well-being.

Tips for Balance: Engage in regular practices that support heart coherence, such as mindful breathing or HeartMath techniques to optimize our heart-brain connection, reduce stress, and enhance overall health. Being mindful of our internal frequency and tuning into the natural rhythms of the earth can further amplify the healing effects of our practices.

NEUROPLASTICITY AND THE POWER OF MIND-BODY PRACTICES

One of the most remarkable breakthroughs in modern neuroscience is the concept of neuroplasticity—the brain's remarkable ability to reorganize and adapt throughout our lives. This concept underscores the dynamic nature of the brain, which can form new neural connections in response to experiences, learning, and environmental changes. Mind-body practices such as acupuncture, yoga, breathing exercises, and aromatherapy have been shown to promote neuroplasticity by influencing neural pathways, supporting cognitive function, and enhancing emotional resilience.

Neuroplasticity is crucial for maintaining mental health and well-being, particularly when dealing with stress, emotional trauma, and aging. The ability of the brain to reorganize itself allows us to adapt to life's challenges, whether that means recovering from trauma, adapting to new life circumstances, or enhancing our capacity for learning and growth. Practices such as yoga and mindfulness meditation facilitate this by engaging the brain in ways that promote growth, healing, re-connection and resilience.

Scientific studies underscore the potential of mind-body practices to enhance cognitive performance, regulate emotional states, and alleviate stress. For example, yoga has been shown to enhance brain function by increasing gray matter density, particularly in areas related to memory and emotional regulation. Similarly, acupuncture has been shown to influence brain activity, reduce anxiety, and improve mood by modulating neuro-chemical activity. Together, these practices help harness the brain's inherent plasticity to foster healing and personal transformation.

MINDFULNESS, MEDITATION, AND THE DEFAULT MODE NETWORK

The study of mindfulness and meditation has uncovered critical insights into the brain's Default Mode Network (DMN)—a system of brain regions that is active when we are not focused on external tasks. The DMN plays a key role in self-referential thinking, mind-wandering, and reflection. While the DMN can contribute to emotional distress and rumination, mindfulness meditation has been shown to modulate its activity, promoting present-moment awareness and reducing the impact of stress and anxiety.

Incorporating mindfulness into our daily routine, particularly through practices such as yoga or breath work, helps to shift the brain from the default state of rumination to a more focused, balanced, and peaceful state. The integration of essential oils into mindfulness practices further enhances the experience by providing a sensory dimension that can deepen the meditative state, regulate emotions, and promote emotional resilience. The use of calming scents, such as lavender or sandalwood, has been shown to activate the brain's limbic system, which is responsible for emotion regulation, creating a holistic sensory experience for emotional balance.

NEUROTRANSMITTERS AND THE ENERGETIC EFFECTS OF AROMATHERAPY ON THE BRAIN

Neurotransmitters, the brain's chemical messengers, play a pivotal role in regulating our mood, energy, and cognitive function. The integration of aromatherapy into mind-body practices has been shown to influence neurotransmitter activity; enhancing serotonin, dopamine, and GABA levels—key chemicals that promote feelings of well-being, happiness, and calm.

Essential oils are powerful tools in this process, influencing the olfactory system, which is directly connected to the brain's limbic (emotional regulation) region. This interaction can trigger neuro-chemical changes that help alleviate stress, reduce anxiety, and even enhance cognitive performance. Scents such as rose, bergamot, and frankincense have been shown to reduce cortisol levels, the hormone associated with stress, while also promoting a sense of peace and mental clarity.

Incorporating essential oils into practices like yoga or meditation can amplify their healing effects, aligning the mind-body connection and nervous system regulation to achieve greater emotional and physiological balance.

STRESS, THE HPA AXIS, AND THE ROLE OF ADAPTOGENS

The HPA axis (Hypothalamic-Pituitary-Adrenal axis) is a complex system that governs the body's response to stress. When under chronic stress, the HPA axis becomes dysregulated, leading to a cascade of negative effects on physical and mental health, including adrenal burnout, immune suppression, and emotional instability.

In both traditional healing systems and modern science, adaptogens are recognized for their ability to help regulate the HPA axis, restore balance, and enhance the body's resilience to stress. Adaptogens are natural substances, such as Eleuthrococcus (Siberian Ginseng), Ashwagandha, Rhodiola, and Tulsi (Holy basil) , that help the body adapt to environmental stressors, supporting the nervous system, immune system, and endocrine function as it responds to stressors.

Studies show that when ingested regularly, adaptogens can help reduce the physiological impact of stress, improve cognitive function, and promote emotional well-being. In addition, practices such as yoga, breath work, and aromatherapy can complement the effects of adaptogens, enhancing the body's ability to cope with stress and restore equilibrium.

CONCLUSION

The integration of ancient wisdom with modern science offers a profound opportunity for healing, growth, and transformation. By understanding how the practices of Chinese medicine, yoga, aromatherapy, and other ancient healing traditions align with neuroscientific findings, we can now "prove" that our mind, body, and spirit are positively affected. From neuroplasticity and adaptogens to mindfulness and heart coherence, these practices not only support our physical health but also cultivate emotional resilience, mental clarity, and spiritual well-being.

As we continue to explore the synergy between ancient traditions and cutting-edge science, we open the door to new possibilities for holistic health, empowering ourselves to heal, grow, and live in alignment with the rhythms of nature. This convergence of wisdom offers us a comprehensive road map for fostering vitality, peace, and well-being, helping us navigate the challenges of modern life with grace and resilience.

6
CREATING SACRED SPACE

"At first you might find that nothing happens there. But if you have a sacred space and use it, eventually something will happen.
Your sacred space is where you find yourself again and again."
- Joseph Campbell

Intentional Living to inspire Harmony, Healing, and Peace

Now that you're well-informed through the lens of Chinese medicine and the five elements, it's not much of a stretch to consider that who and what we surround ourselves with, and how we do so, also plays a significant role in our health, success, and well-being on every level.

Our physical environment is not just a backdrop to our lives, as you can understand from the previous chapters; it is an integral part of our well-being and overall sense of harmony. The spaces we inhabit, whether it's our homes, workplaces, or natural surroundings, have a profound impact on our energy, emotions, and overall quality of life that we experience. The quality of our space can also help or inhibit productivity, goals and health.

According to ancient sciences, the arrangement, design, and energy flow of our surroundings are considered imperative to either support or hinder our physical and mental health, creativity, relationships, success, and overall sense of peace.

By understanding the significance of our physical environment and consciously working to create spaces that nourish and uplift us, we can cultivate an environment that fosters well-being and aligns with our intentions and aspirations, making it easier to reach our goals and dreams.

UNDERSTANDING THE PRINCIPLES OF FENG SHUI AND ITS IMPACT ON ENERGY FLOW

Feng shui is an ancient Chinese practice that seeks to harmonize and optimize the flow of energy, known as "qi," in a given space. Optimizing this flow helps to promote balance, well-being, and prosperity. The character 风 "Feng", conveys the concept of air and energy movement, while 水 "Shui", symbolizes the gentle, fluid nature of qi.

Together, 风水 - "Feng Shui" represents the interplay and balance between the two elements of air and water to create a harmonious living environment.

At its core, Feng Shui recognizes that the arrangement and design of our environments can either enhance or disrupt the natural energy flow, influencing every aspect of our lives. By understanding the principles of Feng Shui, we gain the ability to create spaces that support our physical, emotional, and spiritual well-being.

From the placement of furniture and objects to the use of color and materials, Feng Shui teaches us how to align our spaces with the natural forces of energy, encouraging positive Qi to circulate freely and nourish every aspect of our lives.

By consciously working with the principles of Feng Shui, we can create spaces that feel balanced, inviting, and supportive, allowing us to thrive and live in alignment with our highest potential.

THE INTERCONNECTION BETWEEN OUR LIVING SPACES AND WELL-BEING

Our living spaces are not separate from us; they are extensions of our energy, emotions, and overall well-being. The way we arrange, maintain, and interact with our environment can profoundly influence our mood, mindset, and even our physical health.

Have you ever noticed how simply adding a plant, rearranging furniture, or clearing clutter can completely shift the atmosphere of a room—and how you feel in it? Or how completing a long-overdue home project or organizing a space can bring a sense of clarity and motivation?

Just as our surroundings shape us, we imprint our emotions, experiences, and energy into the spaces we inhabit. A cluttered, disorganized environment can contribute to feelings of stress, stagnation, and overwhelm, while a harmonious, intentional space fosters peace, clarity, and inspiration.

By cultivating an environment that feels nurturing, balanced, and aligned with our energy, we create a sanctuary—a place where we can retreat, recharge, and reconnect with ourselves. In caring for our physical surroundings, we are also tending to our own well-being, forming a sacred relationship between our inner and outer worlds.

ACTIONABLE STEPS FOR SPACE CLEARING

Creating a harmonious and energetically balanced environment can enhance well-being and invite positive energy into your space. It starts with a few simple steps:

1. Set an Intention

Before starting, take a moment to set a clear intention for your space.

Visualize the energy you want to bring in (peace joy, clarity, abundance).

You can say a simple affirmation like: *"I release all stagnant energy and welcome fresh, uplifting vibrations into this space."*

2. De-Clutter and Clean

Remove any unnecessary items that no longer serve you.

Physically clean surfaces, floors, and corners where energy can stagnate.

Open windows to allow fresh air to circulate.

3. Use Sound to Shift Energy

Ring a bell, chime, or Tibetan singing bowl in different areas of your space.

Clap your hands or use rhythmic drumming to break up stagnant energy.

Play mantras, uplifting music, or sacred chants to raise the frequency.

4. Smudge with Sacred Herbs

Burn sage, palo santo, cedar, or sweetgrass to cleanse the energy.

Move through your space, wafting the smoke into corners and doorways.

Say an intention while smudging, such as: *"May this space be filled with light and harmony."*

Ensure proper ventilation to allow negative energy to leave.

5. Work with Crystals and Natural Elements

Place black tourmaline, selenite, or clear quartz in your space for protection and energetic cleansing.

Use Himalayan salt or bowls of water to absorb negative energy.

Add fresh plants or flowers to keep the energy vibrant and alive.

6. Light a Candle or Use Essential Oils

Light a candle to symbolize renewal and illumination.

Diffuse purifying essential oils like lavender, palo santo, or frankincense.

7. Perform a Visualization or Prayer

Close your eyes and imagine golden light filling every corner of the space.

Envision negativity dissolving and being replaced by peace and clarity.

Offer gratitude for the space and the energy shift you've created.

8. Maintain the Energy

Repeat space clearing regularly (weekly, monthly, or as needed).

Stay mindful of your own energy—your emotions and thoughts influence the environment.

Keep your space organized, clean, and filled with things that bring joy and inspiration.

By practicing space clearing regularly, you can create a peaceful, high-vibrational environment that supports your well-being, creativity, and spiritual growth.

HOW TO BA GUA A ROOM: A GUIDE TO FENG SHUI WITH THE BA GUA MAP

In Feng Shui, the Ba Gua (pronounced "bah gwah") is a tool used to assess and optimize the flow of energy (Chi) in a space.

It's an ancient Chinese concept that divides a space into eight areas, each corresponding to a particular aspect of life (e.g. wealth, love, health), and is aligned with one of the five elements (wood, fire, earth, metal, water).

"Ba" means "eight," and "Gua" means "trigram," so the Ba Gua map divides your space into eight trigrams that represent different energies and life areas.

Using the Ba Gua map to "bagua" or "feng shui" a room helps balance the energies in your environment, improving your physical, emotional, and spiritual well-being.

FOLLOW THIS STEP-BY-STEP GUIDE ON HOW TO BA GUA A ROOM TO MAXIMIZE HARMONY AND POSITIVE ENERGY FLOW:

Step 1: Understand the Ba Gua Map

The Ba Gua map is usually represented as a grid with nine sections: the center and the eight surrounding areas. Each section corresponds to an area of life.

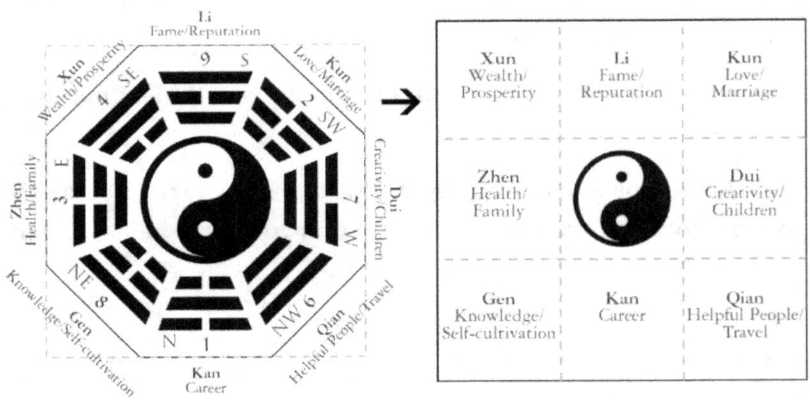

https://www.qcdesignschool.com/2018/03/feng-shui-course-sample-tips-drawing-the-bagua-map/

Step 2: Determine the Layout of the Room

To begin, you need to map the Ba Gua onto your room.

Here's how to do it:

1. **Find the center** of the room. This will correspond to the Health section of the Ba Gua (the center square).
2. **Align the Ba Gua map with the room.** Place the Ba Gua map so that the bottom of the map is aligned with the wall that represents the front door or the entry to the room. You may need to adjust the map slightly to fit your room's layout.
3. **Divide the room into 9 areas** based on the Ba Gua map. You will notice that the room's shape may not perfectly correspond to the square grid, so you'll need to apply the Ba Gua concept in a way that makes sense for the room's layout. The center should always be the heart of the room.

Step 3: Enhance Each Life Area Based on the Ba Gua Map

Once you have the Ba Gua map in place, it's time to enhance each area of your room based on the energies of the corresponding life area. You can add elements, colors, shapes, and items that resonate with each specific area to strengthen the energy flow.

ENHANCEMENTS FOR EACH AREA:

<u>Center (Health)</u>

- **Element:** Earth
- **Colors:** Yellow, brown, beige
- **Shapes:** Square

Enhance with: a grounding object like a ceramic vase, stone sculpture, or crystals. Keep the space tidy and organized.

<u>North (Career & Life Path)</u>

- **Element:** Water
- **Colors:** Black, dark blue
- **Shapes:** Black items or objects with a wavy form

Enhance with: A water fountain, black décor, or a mirror to represent water. This area governs your professional and personal growth, so it's a good place to have motivational objects.

South (Fame & Reputation)

- **Element:** Fire
- **Colors:** Red, bright orange
- **Shapes:** Triangle or pyramidal

Enhance with: Candles, lamps, or red/warm colored art work. This is the area of recognition and social visibility, so adding things that promote warmth and brightness will activate positive energy here.

East (Family & Ancestors)

- **Element:** Wood
- **Colors:** Green, brown
- **Shapes:** Rectangular or tall shapes

Enhance with: Wooden furniture, plants, or family photos. The East represents family health and growth, so introducing greenery or wooden decorations will enhance vitality and harmony.

West (Children & Creativity)

- **Element:** Metal
- **Colors:** White, pastel shades
- **Shapes:** Round or oval shapes

Enhance with: Metal accents, pastel-colored décor, or art that encourages creativity. It's a good place for creative expression, so you could add a creative workspace or artistic elements.

Southeast (Wealth & Abundance)

- **Element:** Wood
- **Colors:** Purple, green, gold

- **Shapes:** Rectangular

Enhance with: Wealth symbols, such as a money tree or abundance jars. Incorporating plants like bamboo, along with green, purple or gold décor can help to attract abundance.

Southwest (Love & Relationships)

- **Element:** Earth
- **Colors:** Pink, peach, earthy tones
- **Shapes:** Square or rectangular

Enhance with: Pairing objects, such as love symbols, pink or red flowers, and soft lighting. This area governs love and partnerships, so romantic touches can elevate the space.

Northeast (Knowledge & Wisdom)

- **Element:** Earth
- **Colors:** Beige, light yellow
- **Shapes:** Square

Enhance with: Bookshelves, study areas, or decorative objects that inspire learning. This is the perfect place for a reading nook or a quiet study area, fostering mental clarity and learning.

Northwest (Helpful People & Travel)

- **Element:** Metal
- **Colors:** White, Grey
- **Shapes:** Circular

Enhance with: Travel memorabilia, objects symbolizing support, or metal items. You can place a compass, travel map, or items from places you've traveled to inspire the flow of helpful energy.

. . .

Step 4: Balance the Elements

As you bagua your room, ensure there is a balance of the five elements (Wood, Fire, Earth, Metal, Water) for the corresponding sections. Each area will benefit from the harmonious presence of these elements, and you can balance them by choosing items that reflect these aspects. For example:

- **Wood** can be represented by plants, wooden furniture, or anything that promotes growth.
- **Fire** can be represented by lighting, candles, or bright colors.
- **Earth** can be represented by grounding objects like stones, pottery, or crystals.
- **Metal** can be represented by metals such as brass, iron, or silver.
- **Water** can be represented by water features, mirrors, or blue tones.

By consciously applying the principles of the Ba Gua map to your room, you create a space that harmonizes with your personal energy and promotes well-being in various aspects of your life.

Remember that Feng Shui is not just about aesthetics—it's about aligning the energy flow in your environment to support your mental, physical, and emotional health. Trust your intuition and find your most aligned flow. If its not your wheelhouse-contact a friend or professional Feng Shui consultant who can help!

PART II
THE POWER OF THE SENSES

Each of our senses—Touch, Smell, Sight, Sound, Taste, and Intuition—serve as a gateway to both outer awareness and inner connection. In Part 2 we explore the wisdom each sense offers, how it corresponds with Chinese Medicine, the elements, practices to support awakening and more...!

7
TOUCH

Touch is not just about physical contact—it is about presence, nourishment, and learning to trust the wisdom of our bodies.

Touch is one of our most profound and transformative senses, serving as a bridge between the physical and emotional realms. It connects us to ourselves, to others, and to the world around us, offering a means of healing that transcends words. Whether through intentional movement, therapeutic bodywork, self-massage, or mindful connection with the elements, touch has the ability to regulate the nervous system, ease emotional distress, and cultivate a deep sense of inner peace. Conversely, when distorted or absent in healthy ways, it can create a disconnect that prevents us from fully experiencing life and being in the present moment.

This chapter explores the science of trauma recovery through the lens of TCM, somatic integration, parts work, Reiki, and Yoga Nidra. By understanding how touch and movement serve as powerful gateways to healing, we can begin to restore a sense of wholeness, safety, and connection—both within ourselves, in our relationships and with the world around us.

When practiced with awareness and intention, movement becomes a form of touch that bridges the physical, energetic, and emotional aspects of being. Therapeutic touch—offered without expectation—can help re pattern negative experiences and restore a sense of trust in the body.

Over the years, I've found that for many individuals, receiving Acupuncture or Reiki was the first time they ever experienced touch as a pure form of support, without demand or obligation. This kind of care can be profoundly transformative, offering a safe and gentle way to reconnect with oneself and the world.

"Trauma is not what happens to us, but what we hold inside in the absence of an empathetic witness."
— Peter A. Levine

How we process our experiences—and the meaning we assign to them—greatly impacts our ability to heal and recover. Trauma, for the sake of clarity in our discussion here, exists along a spectrum, and is unique to each person. It can essentially arise from experiencing *too much, too soon* (such as a sudden car accident or loss) or *too little, too late* (such as neglect in childhood or adulthood).

When we lack the internal or external resources to process these experiences in a healthy, supported way, they often remain unresolved. This can lead to patterns of emotional, mental, and physical distress, even when the original threat is long gone. Trauma, at its core, disrupts our ability to feel safe, grounded, and at home in our own bodies. Because it is experienced through the sensory system—especially the sense of touch—understanding its impact is essential for healing and reclaiming a sense of connection to life.

"In order to stay healthy, our nervous systems and psyches need to face challenges and succeed in meeting them. When this need is not met, or when we are challenged and cannot triumph, we end up lacking vitality and are unable to fully engage in life. Those of us who have been defeated

by war, abuse, accidents, and other traumatic events suffer far more severe consequences."

— Peter A. Levine, *Waking the Tiger: Healing Trauma*

As we begin this exploration of the Six Senses, consider each as a gateway to developing an "empathetic witness" within—a healer and guide toward your own greater freedom and harmony.

TOUCH THROUGH THE LENS OF CHINESE MEDICINE

In Chinese medicine, the sense of touch is deeply connected to the Earth element, which governs nourishment, stability, and our relationship with the physical world. The Spleen and Stomach meridians, responsible for digestion and assimilation, mirror our need for tactile connection—both physically and emotionally.

Just as the Earth provides a foundation for life, touch grounds us, offering comfort, security, and a sense of belonging.

When the Earth element is imbalanced, one may experience physical symptoms like digestive issues or fatigue, as well as emotional disturbances like overthinking, worry, or disconnection. Engaging in touch-based practices such as massage, acupuncture, or mindful movement can strengthen the Earth element, helping to bring balance and deeper felt sense of embodiment.

THE SOMATIC CONNECTION: THERAPEUTIC TOUCH TO INTEGRATE THE MIND AND SPIRIT

The term SOMA refers to the body, especially the intricate relationship between body and mind.

"Somatic" therapies and practices therefore, encourage individuals to tune into and "touch" the sensations, emotions, and stored experiences within the body. Through intentional touch—whether through direct physical modalities, body work or the touch of your own movement or inner awareness—we can access deeper layers of consciousness, uncover repressed emotions, and bring attention to energetic imbalances that may be causing physical or emotional discomfort using these therapies.

The concept of somatic integration is grounded in the belief that the body holds memories of past experiences, and these experiences are often stored in the form of muscle tension, chronic pain, or restricted movement. When trauma occurs, especially after the fact as in PTSD (Post Traumatic Stress Disorder), it can manifest as physical sensations, discomforts, or sensations of numbness in the body as well as disassociation.

Healing from trauma requires integrating these bodily experiences with emotional processing, creating a pathway for the body to reconnect, release, and reclaim the sense of self that has been lost.

"When a young tree is injured it grows around that injury. As the tree continues to develop, the wound becomes relatively small in proportion to the size of the tree. Gnarly burls and misshapen limbs speak of injuries and obstacles encountered through time and overcome. The way a tree grows around its past contributes to its exquisite individuality, character, and beauty. I certainly don't advocate for traumatization to build character, but since trauma is almost a given at some point in our lives, the image of the tree can be a valuable mirror."

— Peter A. Levine,

Waking the Tiger: Healing Trauma

Just as the tree grows around its past to create a beautiful, unique tapestry; we too create our own "tapestries", woven into expression through our bodies and our own connection with physical movement and embodiment. Movement offers a direct way to grow, access and consciously integrate these places of held trauma. In doing so, we claim our own beautiful growth and version of the above metaphor.

Through practices like Qi Gong, Tai Chi, Reiki and Yoga, we intentionally move the body, facilitating energy flow along meridians, Nadis and through Chakras while also allowing for emotional and physical release. These practices encourage the body to "speak" through its sensations, touch, and movements, providing an outlet for deep healing and deeper listening.

BUILDING INNER SAFETY AND CONNECTION THROUGH TOUCH AND MOVEMENT

For those who have experienced trauma, the body can become a place of disconnection and neglect. When traumatic events occur, the physical body may hold onto these experiences, leading to a numb, disassociated or avoidance type of awareness.

Reconnecting with the body through touch—either through movement, body work, or mindful contact—is essential in building inner safety and helping to re-establish that the body can become a safe place again, as well as provide an opportunity to awaken the mind to new possibilities of ways of being.

Somatic practices, such as Somatic Experiencing, Trauma-Sensitive Yoga and Body-Based Therapies, use movement as a gentle, non-invasive form of touch that helps individuals safely reconnect with their bodies. These practices invite the practitioner to slowly reintroduce themselves to their sensations, allowing a self guided and gradual re-calibration in order to experience safety, without overwhelming the nervous system.

Research on somatic integration supports the effectiveness of using movement and touch to heal trauma. *Somatic Experiencing®*, a therapeutic approach developed by Peter Levine, emphasizes tracking physical sensations as a way of processing and releasing trauma from the body.

By tuning into the sensations of touch—whether it's the feeling of the feet on the ground, the sensation of breath in the chest, or the movements in the limbs—we can begin to restore a sense of safety and integration within the body.

In fact, a study published in *The Journal of Trauma & Dissociation* found that *Somatic Experiencing®*, which integrates both physical touch and emotional release, was successful in reducing symptoms of PTSD, especially when combined with body awareness techniques.

Similarly, Trauma-Sensitive Yoga has been shown to improve self-regulation in individuals with PTSD. A study in *The Journal of Alternative and Complementary Medicine* confirmed that yoga's ability to engage the body through mindful movements—while being in touch with sensations—helps regulate the autonomic nervous system, which plays a key role in relaxation and stress recovery.

Through these practices, the body learns to touch and hold *itself* with kindness, fostering a feeling of safety and security that can allow for emotional release, greater resilience and healing.

SIMPLE SOMATIC PRACTICES FOR NERVOUS SYSTEM REGULATION

These SOMA practices help regulate the nervous system by engaging the body's natural ability to restore balance, release tension, and cultivate a sense of safety and well-being. These can be used if feeling caught in fight, flight, freeze or fawn response and are easy to use anytime and in any setting. Try them all and find the ones that help you the most with your present concern or challenge. The "help" they offer will often be felt as a relief, calm or better feeling state.

GROUNDING AND ORIENTATION TECHNIQUES

- **Orienting:** Gently look around your space, naming objects or noticing colors and textures to signal safety to the brain.
- **5-4-3-2-1 Sensory Check-In:** Identify **5 things you can see, 4 things you can touch, 3 things you can hear, 2 things you can smell, and 1 thing you can taste** to ground in the present moment.

- **Feet Awareness:** Place both feet firmly on the ground, noticing the contact points and the support beneath you.
- **Self-Holding:** Cross your arms and place each hand on the opposite shoulder or upper arm, applying gentle pressure to create a sense of containment and safety.

BREATH WORK AND REGULATION

- **Extended Exhale Breathing:** Inhale for **4 counts**, exhale for **6-8 counts** to activate the parasympathetic nervous system.
- **4-7-8 Breathing:** Inhale for **4 counts**, hold for **7 counts**, exhale for **8 counts** to promote relaxation.
- **Sighing Breath:** Take a deep inhale through the nose, then exhale audibly with a sigh, releasing tension.
- **Humming or Vagal Toning:** Humming, chanting, or using a deep "Voo" sound vibrates the vagus nerve, promoting calmness.

WEIGHTED AND SENSORY-BASED PRACTICES

- **Weighted Blanket:** Provides deep pressure stimulation, signaling safety to the nervous system.
- **Body Scan with Weighted Object:** Lay down and place a heavy pillow or book on your chest or abdomen, focusing on the sensation of support.
- **Cold Water Exposure:** Splash cold water on the face or hold an ice cube to engage the dive reflex, which calms the nervous system.
- **Warmth Therapy:** Use a hot shower or bath, heating pad, warm tea, or a hot water bottle to create a sense of security.

MOVEMENT AND RELEASE

- **Shaking (Neurogenic Tremors):** Stand and gently shake your hands, arms, and legs to release stored tension and stress.
- **Rocking Motion:** Gently sway from side to side or rock back and forth while seated to soothe the nervous system.
- **Somatic Hug:** Wrap your arms around yourself and squeeze gently, breathing deeply into the embrace.
- **Butterfly Tapping (Bilateral Stimulation):** Cross your arms over your chest and tap rhythmically, alternating hands.

CONNECTION AND CO-REGULATION

- **Eye Contact and Social Engagement:** Looking at a trusted person, pet, or even a favorite photograph can help regulate the nervous system.
- **Hand on Heart or Belly:** Placing a hand over the heart or abdomen and breathing deeply fosters a sense of comfort.
- **Soft Singing or Chanting:** Singing at a comfortable volume can regulate the vagus nerve and enhance relaxation.
- **Petting an Animal:** The rhythmic motion of petting a cat or dog releases oxytocin and lowers stress hormones.

Refer to *www.traumahealingaccelerated.com* for more information and programs to support your healing with these methods. Also check out *www.theembodylab.com* for more programs and trainings.

SOMATIC MOVEMENT AND MERIDIANS: TOUCHING THE ENERGY FLOW

In Chinese medicine, movement is seen as a vital component in restoring the flow of Qi (pronounced "chee"- or life force energy) through the body's meridians.

Meridians are channels that carry energy throughout the body, and when Qi becomes blocked or stagnant, it can lead to physical pain, illness, and/or emotional disturbances. These energetic blocks are often experienced physically as discomfort or tightness in specific areas of the body.

Touch, through movement and self massage/acupressure can help clear these blocks and encourage the free flow of Qi.

According to a study published in *The Journal of Alternative and Complementary Medicine*, Qi Gong was found to improve circulation, reduce stress, and enhance energy levels. These benefits arise from the mindful movements that stimulate meridians and encourage the free flow of Qi throughout the body.

REIKI- UNIVERSAL LIFE FORCE ENERGY

A Japanese energy healing practice, Reiki (or "Universal Energy"- Ki is the Japanese word for Qi) is a powerful form of therapeutic touch that works to restore balance and harmony within the body, mind, and spirit.

Usui Reiki, founded by Mikao Usui in the early 20th century, is based on the concept of channeling universal life force energy through the hands and inner meridians to offer deep relaxation, emotional healing, and overall well-being to the recipient and the one channeling it. It is always non-harming and benevolent energy that anyone can benefit from. Practitioners use light or hovering touch over the body's energy centers, allowing the Reiki energy to flow intuitively to areas that need healing.

Holy Fire® Reiki, a more recent evolution introduced by William Lee Rand, that incorporates a refined, spiritually guided frequency that enhances self-healing, clarity, and purification at a deep level and operates 24/7.

Holy Fire® Reiki is known for its ability to heal trauma, release energetic blockages, and promote a profound sense of inner peace. Both

Usui and Holy Fire® Reiki are gentle, yet powerful, methods of healing that work beyond the physical body, addressing emotional, mental, and spiritual imbalances. As forms of therapeutic touch, they help gently regulate the nervous system, reduce stress, and create a space for self-healing, self-awareness, renewal, and transformation.

PARTS WORK AND TOUCH: RECONNECTING WITH FRAGMENTED PARTS OF THE SELF

Trauma often leads to this fragmented sense of self, where parts of the body or psyche become disassociated from one another, making it difficult to experience full emotional or physical presence. Touch, in the form of body-based movement, helps foster inner safety, while at the same time, beginning to invite the parts of ourselves to re engage and work together as a whole.

The concept of parts work is grounded in the idea that we all have multiple sub personalities or "parts" within us, developed by psychologist Richard Schwartz. He identified that some of these parts are protective or nurturing, while others may hold onto past trauma, fear, or unresolved emotions as a form of protection or necessary isolation. These fragmented parts often "speak" through patterns of reaction, physical sensations-creating pain, numbness or discomfort in the body, as well as mental patterns of fear, attack and confusion.

Through frameworks such as Internal Family Systems (IFS), parts work focuses on connecting with and healing the wounded or fragmented aspects of the self. By engaging in conscious dialog, individuals can begin to "touch" these fragmented parts and facilitate integration by becoming aware of their job, needs, presence and age.

Emerging research into parts work and somatic integration suggests that combining body-focused practices with psychological therapies, such as IFS, can lead to better emotional regulation and resilience.

A study on somatic integration in PTSD (Post Traumatic Stress Disorder) recovery, published in *The Journal of Traumatic Stress*, showed that integrating body awareness with emotional processing significantly reduced hyper vigilance and dissociation in individuals with PTSD.

A study published in *The Journal of Trauma and Dissociation* found that individuals participating in somatic therapies showed reduced symptoms of PTSD, including lower anxiety, better sleep, and improved emotional regulation. These results were achieved through the mindful practice of movement and therapeutic touch, which engaged the body in a process of rebalancing the nervous system and regaining emotional self-regulation.

Trauma-sensitive yoga, as another example, offers participants a chance to explore their physical boundaries, regulate their breathing, and begin to reclaim a sense of agency in their bodies in a way that honors the needs of a nervous system that is dysregulated, in a way that they are active in re-creating.

TOUCH AND THE HEALING POWER OF YOGA NIDRA

In the context of touch, the subtle yet profound practice of Yoga Nidra, or yogic sleep, emerges as a powerful tool for healing from trauma and regulating the system in general. While touch is often thought of as a physical experience, it also extends to the inner layers of the self—the emotional, mental, and energetic bodies.

Yoga Nidra serves as a gentle yet transformative way to "touch" these deeper aspects of our being, gently and safely, while offering an opportunity for profound relaxation, release, and integration.

Yoga Nidra, as taught by Swami Satyananda Saraswati, is described as "*a state of mind between wakefulness and sleep that opens deep reservoirs of healing within the subconscious and unconscious layers of the mind.*"

In his book *Yoga Nidra*, Swami Satyananda writes: "*By means of Yoga Nidra, the samskaras, the deep impressions which are the driving force behind karma, can be cleared at their root, thereby neutralizing many of the habits, tendencies, and behavioral patterns which dominate our lives.*"

For those healing from trauma, Yoga Nidra offers a safe and supportive space to access and release unresolved emotions and memories stored within the body. Trauma often disrupts our sense of safety, leaving the nervous system dysregulated and the body holding patterns of tension or hyper vigilance.

Through the deeply restorative practice of Yoga Nidra, individuals are guided into a state of complete relaxation where the body can reset, and the mind can reprocess challenging experiences without the risk of overwhelm.

This practice works by activating the parasympathetic nervous system, fostering a sense of safety and calm, and allowing the body's natural healing mechanisms to engage. The practice takes the brain from an Alpha or awake, busy state, into Theta, or deeply relaxed and connected state.

Yoga Nidra can gently address the imprints of trauma (samskaras) by providing a state of awareness that transcends the conscious mind's defenses, enabling integration at the deepest levels and the resolve (Sankalpa) to move beyond them.

The connection to touch lies in the somatic experience of Yoga Nidra. As the practitioner moves through the practice, attention is guided systematically through different parts of the body, often starting with a rotation of consciousness. This body scan serves as a way to reconnect with parts of the body that may have been numbed or disassociated due to trauma, re-establishing a gentle and nurturing relationship with oneself.

For anyone seeking to heal from trauma, Yoga Nidra is a profound complement to other sensory practices. It provides connection to inner or "psychic" touch—a soothing and supportive connection to the self—that bridges the gap between body and mind, offering a pathway to resilience, renewal, and wholeness. It is a reminder that healing is not about forcing change, but rather about allowing the body and mind to gently return to their natural state of balance.

As Swami Satyananda Saraswati wisely said: "*Relaxation does not mean sleep. Relaxation means to be blissfully happy, free of tension and one with your inner self.*"

In this way, Yoga Nidra is both a balm for trauma (and life!) and a bridge back to the self, reconnecting us with the healing power within, at a pace that is acceptable and respectful.

CONCLUSION: THE HEALING JOURNEY THROUGH TOUCH

By practicing embodied movement and somatic awareness, we are reminded that healing *is* a journey of touch—one that reconnects us to our bodies, our emotions, and our deepest sense of self. Through this profound re connection, we unlock the full potential for holistic healing, emotional resilience, and physical vitality.

The integration of mind, body, and spirit through touch and movement allow us to reclaim our health, find peace within, and cultivate a sense of harmony in our lives.

Touch is not just about physical contact—it is about feeling fully present in our own skin, receiving nourishment from the world, and learning to trust the wisdom of our bodies.

As you integrate these practices into your life, may you find comfort, resilience, and a renewed connection to the profound wisdom within your own body and sensations.

8
SMELL

Our sense of smell is one of the most powerful and direct connections to our brain and emotions.

It is intimately linked to the limbic system, the part of the brain responsible for regulating emotions, memory, and certain physiological responses.

What is particularly fascinating is how scent can trigger both immediate and profound changes in our mental and emotional states.

For instance, when a mother smells her newborn baby's head, her olfactory system sends signals to her brain that trigger a cascade of hormones and chemicals necessary for providing nourishment to her child through breastfeeding. The amazing part of this process is that the mother's body adjusts the composition of her breast milk according to the baby's immediate needs—based solely on the scent given off by the child's head!

This is just one example of how aromatics can influence our body's systems in subtle, and powerful ways.

The power of smell extends far beyond maternal bonding; it is central many other processes in life including safety, nourishment and even finding our most compatible mates.

SMELL THROUGH THE LENS OF CHINESE MEDICINE

The sense of smell is governed by the Metal element, which corresponds to the Lungs and Large Intestine meridians and is deeply tied to breath, purification, and the ability to let go.

The breath is our primary link to life force energy (Qi), and aromatic influences can profoundly impact our mood, emotions, and overall health. Inhalation of scents can strengthen or disperse energy in the Lungs, making aromatherapy and breath work powerful tools for maintaining balance.

When the Metal element is deficient or stagnant, one may experience grief, difficulty letting go, or respiratory issues such as congestion or shortness of breath. Engaging with cleansing aromas like eucalyptus, frankincense, or citrus can support the Lung meridian, helping to clear stagnation and invite clarity, vitality, and emotional release.

AROMATHERAPY

The use of essential oils to improve health and well-being through the olfactory sense, is a great way to deliberately influence and support the health of the brain and body.

Over the years, aromatherapy has gained immense recognition, not just for its ability to uplift one's mood but for its remarkable healing potential in balancing emotional health. Aromatherapy offers an incredibly safe, natural, and effective method of supporting the emotional and mental aspects of health, with minimal to no side effects-unlike many pharmaceutical treatments.

AROMATHERAPY FOR EMOTIONAL AND MENTAL HEALTH

Extensive research has been conducted to explore the therapeutic benefits of aromatherapy, particularly in managing emotional and mental health challenges. One area where aromatherapy has shown great promise is in the treatment of Post-Traumatic Stress Disorder (PTSD), as well as anxiety, stress, and depression. Many of the essential oils commonly used in aromatherapy, including lavender, bergamot, vanilla, and frankincense, have been found to reduce anxiety levels, promote relaxation, and support emotional stability.

A study published on the effects of aromatherapy in patients recovering in ICU's highlighted the effectiveness of lavender, Roman chamomile, and neroli oils in reducing anxiety, improving sleep quality, and stabilizing vital signs.

This research illustrated how aromatherapy could not only aid in emotional healing but also in physical recovery. By inhaling these essential oils, patients experienced a calming effect, lowering their anxiety and stress levels while simultaneously improving their sleep quality without the use of traditional medications.

Another study showed significant reductions in anxiety and improvements in sleep quality for patients in intensive care units (ICU) who received aromatherapy treatments. The results were clear: patients who inhaled a blend of essential oils reported lower levels of anxiety, improved blood pressure, and better overall relaxation. The study concluded that aromatherapy could be a powerful and natural tool for promoting healing and emotional well-being, especially in high-stress environments like hospitals and dental offices.

THE AROMA FREEDOM TECHNIQUE: HARNESSING THE HEALING POWER OF SCENT

The Aroma Freedom Technique (AFT) is a specialized protocol that uses the power of essential oils to facilitate emotional release and healing, created by Dr. Benjamin Perkus Ph.D.

AFT acknowledges the profound impact that emotions and thoughts have on our overall well-being, especially on brain health. By using carefully chosen essential oils, AFT works to release emotional blocks, negative thought patterns, and limiting beliefs that may be holding us back mentally and emotionally.

What makes AFT especially powerful is its ability to interact with the limbic system and amygdala, two key areas of the brain involved in memory processing and emotional regulation. The limbic system is highly sensitive to smell, and through AFT, the specific oils used can help reset emotional responses, reduce negative emotions, and promote mental clarity and focus.

For instance, lavender is often used to calm the mind, while citrus oils are known to promote feelings of joy and upliftment. Over time, this practice of AFT can result in profound shifts in how we process emotions, handle stress, and approach life's challenges.

The Aroma Freedom Technique, offers a holistic approach to improving brain function, mental clarity, and emotional well-being by addressing the emotional roots of physical discomfort. It is a simple yet effective tool for those seeking to heal on a deeper level and optimize their cognitive and emotional health.

For more information on AFT, including courses and resources, visit *www.AromaFreedom.com.*

SAFETY AND EFFICACY OF AROMATHERAPY

One of the greatest advantages of aromatherapy is its minimal side effects and ease of use compared to conventional pharmaceutical interventions.

Unlike medications, which can often lead to a variety of adverse reactions, essential oils are a natural, gentle, and non-invasive way to promote healing and emotional balance. While aromatherapy is generally safe, it is important to use essential oils with care due to their potency. Because essential oils are highly concentrated, it is crucial to follow the correct usage guidelines, especially when applying them topically or using them in diffuser.

To ensure safety and effectiveness, always seek high-quality essential oils that are pure and free from synthetic additives. Quality oils are extracted using proper methods, such as steam distillation or cold pressing, ensuring that their therapeutic properties remain intact. It is also important to dilute essential oils before applying them to the skin and to perform a patch test to avoid any allergic reactions or sensitivities.

When using essential oils for emotional support or healing, it's essential to listen to your body. While lavender might be calming for one person, it may not have the same effect on someone else. Experimenting with different oils and observing how they affect your emotions and mental state can help you find the oils that resonate with and help you the most.

HOW TO USE ESSENTIAL OILS SAFELY: KEY TIPS

To safely to avoid adverse reactions, follow these key guidelines for correct use:

1. **Dilute Properly** – Essential oils are highly concentrated and should always be diluted before applying to the skin. A safe dilution ratio is 1-3% (1 drop per teaspoon of carrier oil for sensitive areas, up to 5 drops per teaspoon for general use). Suitable carrier oils include coconut, jojoba, and sweet almond oil.
2. **Perform a Patch Test** – Before applying an essential oil to a large area, do a patch test by diluting a small amount and applying it to the inside of your wrist. Wait 24 hours to check for irritation or allergic reactions.
3. **Avoid Direct Sun Exposure with Citrus Oils** – Certain essential oils, especially citrus oils like **bergamot, lemon, lime, grapefruit, and orange**, are **phototoxic** and can cause

skin burns or irritation when exposed to sunlight. Avoid sun exposure for **12-24 hours** after applying them to your skin.

4. **Do Not Ingest Essential Oils** – Unless advised by a qualified aromatherapist or using an FDA approved source, do not ingest essential oils. They are highly concentrated and can be toxic if consumed improperly. (Young Living Vitality Oils are FDA approved for internal use)
5. **Use Caution During Pregnancy & With Children** – Some essential oils are not safe for pregnant women, nursing mothers, or young children. Oils such as clary sage, rosemary, and cinnamon should be avoided during pregnancy. Always consult a professional before use. For young children, use only child-safe oils in very low dilutions.
6. **Be Mindful of Pets** – Many essential oils, including tea tree, eucalyptus, peppermint, and citrus oils, can be toxic to pets. If diffusing around animals, ensure they have access to fresh air and observe for any signs of distress.
7. **Use a Diffuser Safely** – When diffusing essential oils, limit sessions to 30-60 minutes at a time and ensure proper ventilation. Continuous diffusion can overwhelm the nervous system and cause sensitivity or irritation.
8. **Store Properly** – Keep essential oils in dark glass bottles away from direct sunlight, heat, and moisture. Proper storage preserves their potency and prevents oxidation, which can lead to skin irritation.
9. **Avoid Applying Near Eyes, Ears, and Mucous Membranes** – Essential oils should never be applied directly to sensitive areas like the eyes, inside the ears, or open wounds. If irritation occurs, do not rinse with water—instead, apply a carrier oil like jojoba or olive oil to dilute and soothe the affected area.
10. **Know Your Body's Sensitivity** – If you have asthma, allergies, or sensitive skin, introduce essential oils gradually and in low concentrations to avoid adverse reactions. Discontinue use immediately if any discomfort occurs.

By following these safety guidelines, you can enjoy the benefits of essential oils while minimizing risks, ensuring a safe and enjoyable aromatherapy experience.

PURITY AND PRODUCT QUALITY

The purity of essential oils is crucial for ensuring their therapeutic potential. Only high-quality, pure essential oils should be used for aromatherapy.

Essential oils that are adulterated with chemicals or other substances may not have the desired effect and could even cause harm. To ensure you are using the best possible oils, seek reputable brands that provide detailed information on sourcing, testing, and purity standards.

I use only Young Living Essential Oils as they offer the highest quality standard of testing in the industry and I love how they honor a Seed to Seal process with all that they make and grow on their own farms. Quality is especially important if you wish to use essential oils for ingestion such as YL's "Vitality" line, made for ingestion and FDA approved for that use or for therapeutic processes such as AFT, in which you are deeply inhaling aromas directly into the brain.

Visit *www.youngliving.com* for more information and how to safely use Essential Oils for therapeutic use.

CONCLUSION: THE TRANSFORMATIVE POTENTIAL OF AROMATHERAPY

Aromatherapy, with its deeply rooted connection to our sense of smell, offers a safe, natural, and effective way to promote emotional well-being and support mental health. Its potential to enhance mood, reduce anxiety, improve sleep, and promote relaxation has been proven by decades of research. Unlike pharmaceutical treatments, aromatherapy works with the body's own healing systems, offering a gentler approach with far fewer side effects.

By using essential oils mindfully and responsibly, we can unlock their transformative power to promote emotional healing, increase mental clarity, and restore balance to the body and mind. Whether through traditional practices of Aromatherapeutic use or modern techniques like the Aroma Freedom Technique, the power of smell can be a powerful tool for healing and self-discovery.

With a deeper understanding of how essential oils interact with the brain and body, we can fully embrace the healing potential of aromatherapy and use it to enhance our emotional health, cultivate inner peace, and thrive in a world that constantly challenges our mental and emotional resilience.

9
SIGHT

Our sense of sight is one of our most cherished gifts, allowing us to experience the vivid beauty and complexity of the world around us.

Sight is more than just a physical ability to perceive light and color; it is a powerful channel for connection, understanding, and transformation. From the awe-inspiring grandeur of a sunset to the subtle details of a loved one's expression, our eyes serve as windows to both the external world and our inner landscapes.

But sight also goes beyond the literal vision—it encompasses the ability to "see" inwardly with clarity, insight, and intuition. It allows us to witness beauty, understand patterns, and find meaning in the world and within ourselves.

As William Shakespeare famously said-*"The Eyes are the windows to your soul."*

THE PHYSIOLOGY OF SIGHT AND ITS CONNECTION TO THE MIND

Our sense of sight is deeply intertwined with the brain, making it a vital component of how we process and interpret reality. The eye itself is an extraordinary organ, capable of detecting light, depth, and color in ways that allow us to navigate the world with precision.

However, sight doesn't end with the eyes—it extends into the mind, where visual information is processed, interpreted, and given meaning.

Modern neuroscience has shown that what we see is influenced by more than just external stimuli; it is shaped by our emotions, memories, and beliefs.

In this way, sight is both physical and psychological. This duality allows us to not only perceive the world as it is but also to create and recreate meaning based on our inner state of perception.

SIGHT THROUGH THE LENS OF CHINESE MEDICINE

In Chinese medicine, sight is associated with the Liver and its paired organ, the Gallbladder, which is governed by the Wood element. The Liver is said to "open into the eyes," meaning that its health is reflected in our ability to see clearly—both physically and metaphorically. When the Liver Qi flows freely, our vision is sharp, and our capacity for foresight, creativity, and decision-making are enhanced. When Liver Qi is stagnant, we may experience blurry vision, irritability, red eyes, or an inability to see possibilities in our lives.

The eyes also reflect the emotional state of the heart and soul. The Chinese term "Shen" (Spirit of the Heart) refers to the spirit or consciousness that can be seen in the brightness and vitality of someone's eyes.

Clear, radiant eyes are seen as a sign of emotional well-being and inner harmony.

THE SYMBOLISM OF SIGHT

Sight has long been considered a metaphor for insight, wisdom, and awareness in many cultures. Expressions like "seeing the bigger picture" or "opening your eyes" to the truth of the matter, remind us that sight extends beyond the physical and into the realms of perception and understanding. It is tied to clarity, discernment, and vision—not just about the world but of our purpose and path.

In spiritual practices, sight is often linked to the Third Eye Chakra, located between the eyebrows and inward toward the top of the spine. This energetic center is associated with intuition, inner wisdom, and the ability to see beyond physical reality. By nurturing our inner vision, we gain access to deeper truths and align ourselves with our highest potential.

THE ROLE OF SIGHT IN DAILY LIFE

In our fast-paced, modern world, it's easy to take the sense of sight for granted. Screens, artificial lighting, and over stimulation can dull our ability to truly "see". Yet, by pausing and paying attention, we can rediscover the power of sight as a tool for mindfulness, connection, and awe.

When we engage our sight intentionally, we begin to notice the small wonders of life—the intricate patterns on a leaf, the play of light and shadow, the emotions in someone's eyes.

This practice of seeing with awareness not only enriches our daily experience but also deepens our appreciation for the beauty that surrounds us.

PRACTICES TO STRENGTHEN AND HONOR SIGHT

Eye Yoga and Exercises

Just as we strengthen other parts of our body, we can nurture and relax our eyes through specific exercises:

- **Palming:** Rub your hands together to generate warmth, then place them gently over your closed eyes. Allow the darkness to relax your vision.
- **Eye Rotations:** Gently move your eyes in a circular motion—clockwise, then counterclockwise, side to side and up and down—to release tension and improve flexibility of the eye muscles.
- **Focus Shifting:** Alternate your focus between near and far objects to reduce eye strain, especially if you spend long hours looking at screens.

NATURE WALKS

Spend time observing the colors, shapes, and textures in nature. The vibrant greens of leaves, the patterns of bark, and the hues of the sky can help refresh tired eyes and calm the mind.

Practice opening your eyes extra wide to take in more beauty!

COLOR THERAPY

Each color in the spectrum carries its own frequency and can affect the mind and body in unique ways.

For example:

- **Green** is calming and restorative.
- **Blue** is soothing and promotes relaxation.
- **Yellow** energizes and stimulates creativity.
- **Red/orange-red and orange** stimulate appetite and energy.

MEDITATION FOR THE THIRD EYE

Close your eyes and focus your attention on the space between your eyebrows. Visualize a glowing indigo or white light expanding with each breath. Practice on this helps to sharpen your intuition and connect you to your inner vision, your inner “flashlight”.

AROMATHERAPY FOR SIGHT AND FOCUS

Essential oils can also support clarity and vision:

- **Rosemary:** Improves mental focus and enhances clarity.
- **Frankincense:** Calms the mind and supports introspection.
- **Peppermint:** Refreshes and stimulates, clears mental fog.
- **Chamomile:** Soothes tired eyes and promotes relaxation.

THE HEALING POWER OF SEEING BEAUTY

There is healing in simply noticing and appreciating beauty. When we allow ourselves to truly see the world—not through the lens of distraction but with open and receptive eyes—we reconnect with the sacredness of life and its ever-present beauty.

A sunrise, a smile, or even the intricate details of a flower can awaken our sense of wonder and inspire a sense of peace and interconnectedness.

Engaging with the beauty around us also teaches us gratitude. As we become more attuned to the small details and quiet moments, we find that the world is always offering us opportunities to see joy, hope, and connection. An experience that often results in deep appreciation for how precious life really is.

Growing up in New Mexico and Arizona, I was fortunate to get to know and be friends with Native peoples of many tribes. Those relationships helped me to learn about the Native American culture where I lived and gave me a deep sense of awe and appreciation for who we really are as human beings on this planet. I feel fortunate to have attended many sacred dances, lodges and ceremonies through my life, since I was a child.

The Navajo or Diné nation of people from the Southwestern US, have a beautiful way of seeing life and the world, which translates to the "Beauty Way".

For me this prayer and the influence of Native peoples have fostered a deep appreciation for this way of life and being in the world. My sincere respect and gratitude.

Here is the Prayer translated into English:

"In beauty I walk
With beauty before me I walk
With beauty behind me I walk
With beauty above me I walk
With beauty around me I walk
It has become beauty again
It has become beauty again
It has become beauty again
It has become beauty again"

As this prayer speaks to, sight is more than observation—it is participation. When we look at the world with intention and curiosity, we engage with it more fully. Whether it's through the practice of mindfulness, the study of art, the intentional act of creating something beautiful or a simple walk in nature, sight becomes a gateway to presence, helping us find balance in the here and now.

By nurturing our physical eyes, cultivating our inner vision, and learning to see with both clarity and compassion, we align ourselves with a deeper truth: the interconnectedness of all things.

Through this practice of "seeing", we discover not only the beauty of the world around us but also the light and beauty within ourselves.

8 TYPES OF COLOR THERAPY AND THEIR SEASONAL QUALITIES

Just as each season has its own energy, each color has its own therapeutic benefits, influencing our senses and emotions in different ways.

Here's how you can use colors to align with the seasons and support your well-being:

Bring in the Calm with Blue (Winter)

Blue, the color of the winter sky and frozen lakes, is renowned for its calming properties. It reduces stress, promotes tranquility, and aids in sleep. Lighter shades of blue are ideal for bedrooms and spaces where relaxation is a priority.

Boost Your Cheer with Yellow (Summer)

Yellow, like the bright summer sun, is associated with happiness and mental clarity. This uplifting color stimulates the mind and enhances concentration, making it ideal for work spaces and study areas where creativity and focus are needed.

Make a Healing, Tranquil Space with Green (Spring)

Green symbolizes the fresh start and growth of spring. This color embodies balance, renewal, and harmony and is known for its calming and healing qualities. Use green in living spaces or relaxation areas to create a sense of peace and rejuvenation.

Get Motivated with a Dab of Red (Late Summer)

Red, the color of fall harvests and cozy warmth, is energizing and stimulating. It increases circulation and motivation. While red should be used sparingly due to its strong influence, it's perfect for exercise spaces or areas where you need a burst of energy to inspire action.

Stimulate Your Creativity with Orange (Autumn)

Orange, a blend of the energetic qualities of red and the uplifting energy of yellow, boosts creativity and mood. Use it in art studios or dining rooms to stimulate appetite and creativity. Its warm tones mirror the energy of autumn, a time for creativity and harvest.

Soothe and Meditate with Purple (Winter)

Purple, particularly lavender, is a color associated with spirituality and relaxation. It has a soothing effect on the mind and is perfect for meditation spaces, just as the quiet stillness of winter invites introspection and deep calm.

Nurture Yourself with Pink (Spring)

Pink, the color of spring blossoms, represents nurturing and love. It has a calming, reassuring effect and is often used in spaces where relaxation and comfort are key. Soft pinks help create an environment of care and self-compassion, mirroring the nurturing spirit of spring.

Make Space for Focus with White (All Seasons)

White, the color of clarity and purity, represents the freshness of snow in winter or the brightness of a new spring day. It symbolizes simplicity and calm and is perfect for spaces that require focus and clarity, such as offices or meditation rooms.

Practicing color therapy in your daily life is a simple yet transformative process. Just like each season affects our senses, being mindful of the colors around us can help us align our energy with our own needs and environment.

Conclusion: The Gift of Sight

Our sense of sight is more than just a way to navigate the world—it is a gateway to clarity, vision, and understanding, both externally and within. Through the lens of Chinese medicine, we recognize how the Wood element and the health of the Liver influence not only our physical eyesight but also our ability to see with wisdom, perspective, and intention. When we nourish our vision—through mindful practices, balancing movement, and deep inner reflection—we cultivate the ability to perceive life with greater awareness and purpose. Sight is not just about what is in front of us; it is about seeing the bigger picture, envisioning new possibilities, and opening ourselves to the beauty and transformation that each season brings.

By honoring and tending to this precious sense, we allow ourselves to live with clarity, adaptability, and a renewed sense of purpose.

10
SOUND

The healing power of sound is as ancient as human civilization itself, woven into the rituals, traditions, and spiritual practices of cultures across the globe.

From the rhythmic drumming of indigenous tribes to the melodic chanting of Vedic mantras in India, sound has been used as a bridge to connect the physical and spiritual realms for as long as humans have existed.

Ancient Egyptians employed vocal toning in their healing temples, while the Greeks, notably Pythagoras, explored the therapeutic effects of harmonic frequencies. Tibetan monks have long utilized singing bowls and overtone chanting to foster meditation and balance, while Gregorian chants in Christian traditions aimed to elevate the soul and bring spiritual harmony.

Modern research echoes this ancient wisdom, revealing the profound impact of sound on the human nervous system, emotions, and energy centers. Techniques such as sound baths, binaural beats, and vibration therapy now merge ancient practices with contemporary science, demonstrating that sound, whether through song, chant, or resonance, remains a timeless and universal tool for healing, alignment, and transformation through frequency shifts.

SOUND THROUGH THE LENS OF CHINESE MEDICINE

The sense of sound is associated with the Water element, which governs the Kidneys and Urinary Bladder meridians and represents wisdom, depth, and our ability to listen—both externally and internally.

In Chinese medicine, the Kidneys are considered the storehouse of Jing (life essence/"savings account") and play a vital role in our longevity, willpower, and the regulation of fear.

Sound, whether through music, chanting, or vibration-based healing, can harmonize the Water element, restoring a sense of calm and equilibrium.

When the Water element is depleted, one may experience tinnitus (ringing in the ears), hearing loss, adrenal fatigue, or deep-seated fear and anxiety. Engaging in toning practices, mantra chanting, sound baths, or simply listening to the sounds of flowing water can replenish Kidney Qi, soothe the nervous system, and enhance deep inner listening, strengthening both intuition and resilience.

Let's explore some sound-based therapies and their affects, with a focus on the scientific and spiritual foundations.

BI-NEURAL BEATS: SYNCHRONIZING THE BRAIN AND BODY

Bi-neural beats occur when two slightly different frequencies are played in each ear, creating a perceived third frequency — the difference between the two. The brain synchronizes its brainwaves to this perceived frequency, a phenomenon known as *brainwave entrainment*.

Bi-neural beats are used for various therapeutic purposes, depending on the frequency of the beats.

- **Alpha Waves (8–12 Hz):** These frequencies are linked to relaxation and stress reduction, helping the mind to remain calm and focused. They are ideal for light meditation or unwinding after a long day, much like the gentle tones of early spring that encourage growth and renewal.
- **Theta Waves (4–8 Hz):** Often associated with deep meditation and creativity, these frequencies facilitate emotional healing and spiritual growth. Theta waves can help you access deeper subconscious levels, much like the quiet stillness of winter, aiding in introspection.
- **Delta Waves (0.5–4 Hz):** Known for their deep connection to restorative sleep, delta waves promote the body's ability to heal and rejuvenate. Listening to delta waves mimics the deep slumber of a winter night, where the body regenerates and restores.

Bi-neural beats can reduce anxiety, improve sleep, enhance creativity, and even alleviate pain. The brain's ability to entrain to these rhythms has been extensively studied, showing significant benefits for mental and physical health.

MANTRA: VIBRATIONAL HEALING AND SPIRITUAL CONNECTION

Mantras are sacred words, sounds, or syllables that are repeated either silently or aloud. These vibrational patterns have long been used in spiritual and healing practices to focus the mind, alleviate stress, and create a deeper connection to the divine. The sound vibrations of mantras resonate with different energy centers (Chakras) in the body, fostering balance and harmony.

- The most well known seed mantra, **Om (AUM)**, is considered the primordial sound of the universe, believed to align the individual with universal consciousness. Repeating "Om" connects you to a sense of unity and inner peace, especially in moments of meditation or spiritual practice.

- Sanskrit mantras, such as "So Hum" or "Ham So," are also commonly used in meditation for deep meditation, aiding practitioners in their journey toward self-realization and connection to higher consciousness through the central channels of the body.

Research on mantra chanting shows that it activates the parasympathetic nervous system, reducing stress and promoting a state of relaxation and peace. Like the rhythmic sound of nature, mantras create a calming environment that helps quiet the mind.

SOLFEGGIO FREQUENCIES: THE ANCIENT HEALING CODES

The Solfeggio frequencies are a set of nine tones derived from the Solfeggio scale, an ancient musical scale believed to have been used in Gregorian chants. These frequencies are considered to have specific healing properties that resonate with different parts of the body, mind, and spirit.

- **396 Hz** – Liberating Guilt and Fear: This frequency helps release negative emotions and limiting beliefs, creating space for personal transformation.
- **417 Hz** – Undoing Situations and Facilitating Change: It is believed to help clear past trauma and facilitate emotional healing, encouraging renewal and hope.
- **528 Hz** – Transformation and Miracles (DNA Repair): Often called the "love frequency," this tone is believed to promote healing at a cellular level, offering a deep sense of inner peace and connection.
- **639 Hz** – Connecting Relationships: This frequency is thought to enhance communication and harmony, promoting emotional healing and interpersonal connections.

- **741 Hz** – Awakening Intuition: It stimulates mental clarity and aids in emotional detoxification, fostering deeper insight and intuition.
- **852 Hz** – Returning to Spiritual Order: This frequency is used to enhance spiritual awareness, clarity, and connection to higher consciousness.

Listening to these frequencies through sound therapy or meditation is believed to realign the body's energy and restore balance, just as different colors or sounds in nature are thought to promote healing in specific ways.

SACRED MUSIC: THE SOUND OF THE DIVINE

Sacred music is often used in spiritual practices to elevate the mind and spirit. It encompasses various forms of music used in different cultures and religions, from Gregorian chants to Indian bhajans and native drumming ceremonies. Sacred music is created with the intention of connecting the listener to divine energies, healing the soul, and promoting inner peace.

- **Gregorian Chants:** These hauntingly beautiful melodies have been used for centuries in Christian monastic traditions. The slow, meditative tones have a calming effect, helping to bring the listener into a state of deep relaxation and spiritual connection.
- **Kirtan:** In Yoga, the practice of chanting devotional songs and mantras (called kirtan) can bring about a sense of unity, peace, and spiritual awakening. These chants often involve rhythmic clapping and the use of instruments, encouraging participants to feel a profound connection to the divine within themselves and others.
- **Tuning Forks and Singing Bowls:** Frequently used in sound healing practices, where specific frequencies are emitted in order to harmonize the body's energy and promote healing.

> The resonance created by these instruments is deeply relaxing, much like the stillness of a sacred space.

Sacred music's power to heal lies in its ability to evoke deep emotional responses, connect individuals to higher spiritual realms, and promote harmony in both the body and mind.

Research has shown that listening to sacred music can reduce stress, lower blood pressure, improve mental functioning and induce a meditative state, fostering healing on a physical, mental, and spiritual level.

SOUND BATHS: IMMERSING THE BODY IN HEALING SOUND

A sound bath is a therapeutic practice in which an individual is relaxing, immersed in a bath of sound waves, typically created using instruments like singing bowls, gongs, and chimes. The frequencies emitted by these instruments flood the body, inducing deep relaxation and promoting emotional and physical healing.

- The healing power of a sound bath is rooted in the concept of vibrational medicine, where the sounds and frequencies are utilized to penetrate the body and balance its energy field.
- A sound bath can help reduce stress, promote mental clarity, enhance creativity, and relieve physical pain. Just as the stillness of nature's sounds can clear the mind, a sound bath encourages the body to release tension and restore balance.

Sound baths are increasingly used in wellness centers and therapeutic settings as a way to promote relaxation and healing. Research suggests that the frequencies in sound baths help reduce cortisol levels, lower heart rate, and enhance the body's natural healing abilities.

SILENCE: THE HEALING FREQUENCY OF SILENCE

Although sound is powerful, silence can be equally therapeutic. Intentional silence offers a special opportunity for deep introspection, relaxation, and mental clarity. It allows the mind to rest and reset, creating space for healing. Especially for the modern day householder, silence can literally be "golden" in its value for maintaining health and balance.

Mindfulness meditation, which often involves quieting the mind through silence, has been shown to reduce stress and anxiety, enhance focus, and improve overall well-being. Silence gives the mind room to process emotions, make sense of experiences, and find peace within.

Research on solitude and quiet environments shows that regular exposure to silence can lead to improved concentration, creativity, and cognitive function. It can also lower blood pressure and promote a sense of calm.

Silence is not simply the absence of sound—it's an intentional practice of stillness, offering the mind and body space to rejuvenate and heal.

CONCLUSION: THE HEALING POWER OF SOUND

Sound—whether through bi-neural beats, mantras, Solfeggio frequencies, sacred music, sound baths, or even silence—is a powerful tool for healing and transformation.

Each type of sound works on different levels, from deep emotional healing to physical restoration, offering us the chance to realign ourselves with the natural rhythms of the universe. By consciously incorporating sound into our daily practices, we can enhance our well-being, reduce stress, improve sleep, and promote emotional and spiritual growth. Whether you're using sound for relaxation, meditation, or physical healing, it is a profound and gentle resource for those seeking balance and requires very little effort to incorporate.

11
TASTE

Taste is not just a necessary sensory experience—it is also a vital aspect of our health.

In Chinese medicine, food is viewed as medicine, and the flavors we consume are believed to have deep effects on our physical, emotional, and spiritual well-being.

Each of the five primary tastes—sour, bitter, sweet, salty, and umami—corresponds to different organ systems in the body and different seasons of the year, creating a profound connection between food, healing, and the natural world.

THE DEEP CONNECTION BETWEEN TASTE AND SMELL

Taste and smell are intimately linked, working together to shape our sensory experiences of food, memory, and emotion. While taste allows us to detect basic flavors—sweet, sour, salty, bitter, and umami—smell provides the complexity and depth that give food its full character. Without the sense of smell, our ability to perceive nuanced flavors diminishes significantly.

This connection is due to the way our brain processes sensory input. When we eat, aromatic compounds travel from the food in our mouths to the olfactory receptors in the nasal cavity. This process, known as *retronasal olfaction*, allows us to detect intricate flavors beyond what our taste buds alone can perceive.

For example, the taste of a ripe strawberry is not just sweet—it carries floral and fruity notes that come from its scent. If you've ever noticed how food tastes bland when you have a cold, it's because your sense of smell is compromised, limiting your ability to fully experience flavor.

Beyond food, the link between taste and smell plays a crucial role in emotional and psychological responses. Smell has a direct connection to the limbic system, the part of the brain responsible for emotions and memory. This is why a familiar scent, like cinnamon or fresh basil, can instantly transport us to childhood moments or specific cultural traditions. Similarly, our cravings and food preferences are influenced by both sensory experiences—certain scents can make us hungry, while others can evoke comfort, nostalgia, or even aversion.

From a holistic health perspective, honoring the connection between taste and smell can enhance mindfulness in eating, deepen our appreciation of seasonal foods, and support emotional well-being.

By engaging both senses fully—savoring the aroma of freshly brewed tea before taking a sip or pausing to inhale the scent of a meal before tasting—we can enrich our sensory experience and strengthen our connection to the present moment.

TASTE THROUGH THE LENS OF CHINESE MEDICINE

Taste is intrinsically linked to the Fire element, which is associated with the Heart and Small Intestine meridians and plays a crucial role in our emotions, digestion, and joy. The different flavors—bitter, sweet, sour, pungent, and salty—each have unique energetic properties that influence various organ systems and functions.

Bitter foods, for instance, help clear heat and support the Heart, while sweet foods nourish the Spleen and provide grounding energy.

When taste is imbalanced, cravings, digestive issues, or emotional highs and lows may arise. Chinese medicine encourages mindful eating and the consumption of a variety of seasonal foods to maintain harmony between the elements, ensuring that our meals both nourish and balance our physical and emotional well-being.

THE ART OF BALANCE IN COOKING AND HEALTH

In the Netflix series *Salt, Fat, Acid, Heat* (and her book of the same name), Samin Nosrat masterfully explores how these four essential elements shape the foundation of cooking. Her approach highlights the delicate balance of flavors and textures that elevate a dish—an insight that also aligns beautifully with the principles of Chinese dietary therapy.

I was particularly drawn to how she presented the sensory experience of food in such a visually stunning and enticing way. Watching her work deepened my appreciation for taste and food chemistry, leading to more flavorful and satisfying meals in my own kitchen (as confirmed by my very happy husband!).

Naturally, this made me think about the connection between food, flavor, and our organ systems from a Chinese medicine perspective.

The way we balance salt, fat, acidity, and heat in a dish mirrors how we can balance our bodies through seasonal eating and mindful nourishment.

In this chapter, we'll explore how an understanding of these foundational elements—both in cooking and holistic health—can enhance not just the flavors in your meals, but also your overall health and well-being.

SWEET: NOURISHING THE SPLEEN AND STOMACH – SPRING AND LATE SUMMER

Flavor Profile

Sweet flavors are the most commonly recognized and cherished in our diet. In Chinese medicine, the sweet taste is associated with the Spleen and Stomach, the organs responsible for digestion and nourishment. Sweetness is naturally calming and restorative, promoting energy production and blood circulation. However, the key is balance —excessive sweetness can lead to dampness in the body, resulting in sluggish digestion, mental fog and mucus, weak muscles and weight gain.

Seasons for Sweet: Spring and Late Summer

- **Spring:** This is a time for renewal, growth, and the expansion of energy. The liver is most active during this season, and sweet foods support the liver by nourishing the body's energy reserves and aiding digestion. Think of the naturally sweet foods of spring, like young greens, carrots, beets, and sprouted grains. These light, sweet foods help cleanse the body after the winter months.
- **Late Summer:** This season, which is a transition between summer and autumn, corresponds to the Earth element in Chinese medicine and is linked to the Spleen and Stomach. It is a time for strengthening the body's core energy, and sweet foods can help to stabilize energy levels and provide nourishment. Seasonal fruits like peaches, plums, and berries can be enjoyed in moderation to support the body's needs.

Health Benefits: Sweet foods, such as squash, carrots, and root vegetables, help to tone the stomach and spleen and are believed to generate blood and help in the production of vital energy (Qi). In addition, they help to promote a sense of grounding and warmth, which is especially needed during the transitions between seasons.

Example from *Salt, Fat, Acid, Heat*: In the episode on **Acid**, Samin Nosrat demonstrates how a small amount of sweetness—like the addition of honey or sugar—balances acidic dishes. The same principle applies to Chinese medicine, where sweetness helps to moderate the sour and bitter flavors that are often more pungent in certain seasonal foods. A roasted butternut squash soup with a touch of honey or maple syrup is a perfect example of balancing sweet flavors for health.

SOUR- DETOXIFYING LIVER/GALL BLADDER- SPRING AND SUMMER

Flavor Profile:

The sour taste is invigorating and is believed to help promote the flow of Qi and stimulate digestion. Sour foods are connected with the Liver, which is responsible for the smooth flow of energy throughout the body. In Chinese medicine, the liver is particularly associated with emotional balance, and sour flavors are believed to help resolve stagnation, and especially help to regulate emotional blockages such as anger and frustration.

Seasons for Sour: Spring and Summer

- **Spring:** Sour flavors help invigorate and detoxify the body, which is essential during the spring, a time of renewal and growth. Foods like citrus fruits (lemons, limes, and oranges), sour plums, and vinegars are excellent choices. These help support the liver's cleansing processes and stimulate bile production, which is crucial for digestion.
- **Summer:** As the season of abundance and outward activity, summer requires the cooling and detoxifying effects of sour flavors. Sour vegetables, fermented foods (such as kimchi or sauerkraut), and vinegar-based dishes are particularly beneficial. These help to break down heat and dampness in the body, cooling down the excess warmth that can accumulate in the summer.

Health Benefits: Sour foods stimulate digestive juices and liver function, which is important for detoxifying and clearing excess heat or stagnation from the body. Additionally, they support the body's natural detox processes and can help promote healthier skin, a common issue in the summer months.

Example from *Salt, Fat, Acid, Heat*: The **Acid** episode is key for understanding the importance of sourness in balance. The tangy quality of vinegar, or the sharpness of a squeeze of lemon, can transform a dish from being flat to complex and well-rounded. In Chinese medicine, incorporating sour elements like citrus or pickles with fresh greens balances the liver's Qi and is perfect for a healthy, detoxifying spring or summer meal.

BITTER: CLEARING HEAT AND DRYNESS – SUMMER AND AUTUMN

Flavor Profile

The bitter taste is known for its cooling and drying properties. In Chinese medicine, the Heart and Small Intestine are the organs associated. Bitters are thought to clear heat and dryness from the body, making them essential for maintaining balance during the hot summer months and the dry, crisp air of autumn.

Seasons for Bitter: Summer and Autumn

- **Summer:** Bitter flavors help to clear excess heat from the body, which is abundant during the hot summer months. Foods like bitter melon, dandelion greens, and arugula are perfect for cooling the body and alleviating heat buildup.
- **Autumn:** As the weather begins to dry and cool, bitter foods help to clear excess heat from the body, especially in the lungs and digestive system. They also support the body's transition to the more introspective energies of fall. Foods like endive, kale, and bitter greens support lung health, which is crucial in autumn.

Health Benefits: Bitter foods help clear excess heat and toxicity from the body, particularly in the digestive system and skin. They also help to prevent dryness, keeping the body's moisture levels balanced, especially during the dry autumn months.

Example from *Salt, Fat, Acid, Heat*: In the **Salt** episode, Nosrat emphasizes the importance of balancing salty flavors, but bitter flavors also come into play for cooling down rich or fatty dishes. A bitter green salad, such as one with arugula, pairs wonderfully with a rich, fatty dressing to balance out the heaviness, promoting digestive health and cleansing the system.

SALTY: SUPPORTING THE KIDNEYS – WINTER

Flavor Profile

Salty foods have an important role in balancing the Kidneys, the organs associated with water, fluid balance, and vitality. In Chinese medicine, the kidneys are considered the foundation of life, and their energy supports growth, reproduction, and longevity. The salty flavor is considered grounding, stabilizing, and vital for maintaining water balance in the body.

Season for Salty: Winter

- **Winter:** Winter is the season associated with the Kidneys, and salty flavors are crucial for supporting the body's deep reserves. Salty foods like seaweed, miso, and salted fish are excellent choices for this time of year, as they nourish the kidneys, strengthen the bones, and promote warmth and vitality.
- **Health Benefits:** Salty foods help to nourish the kidneys, improve hydration, and support overall energy levels during the colder months. They also enhance the body's ability to retain moisture, prevent dryness, and balance fluids in the body.

Example from *Salt, Fat, Acid, Heat*: In the **Fat** episode, the importance of fat in cooking is explored, but salt is also a crucial balancing agent. Adding salt to rich, fatty foods not only enhances the flavor but also provides the necessary grounding and nourishment that the kidneys require during the winter. A warming bowl of miso soup, rich in salt and fat, is a perfect example of winter food that nurtures the body and balances energy.

UMAMI: THE FIFTH TASTE – BALANCING ALL SYSTEMS

Flavor Profile

Umami, the savory taste often associated with foods like mushrooms, soy sauce, and aged cheeses, is believed to enhance the overall flavor profile of a dish while promoting a sense of fullness and satisfaction. In Chinese medicine, umami is linked to the Stomach and Spleen and is thought to enhance digestion and increase energy.

Seasons for Umami: Throughout the Year

- **All Seasons:** Umami is considered a balancing flavor that can be used throughout the year. It nourishes the digestive system and harmonizes the other flavors. Foods like miso, seaweed, tomatoes, and fermented soy products (such as soy sauce) are rich in umami and can be incorporated into dishes year-round.
- **Health Benefits:** Umami is thought to boost metabolism, improve digestion, and enhance the absorption of nutrients. It also promotes a sense of satisfaction, preventing overeating and encouraging balanced meals.

Example from *Salt, Fat, Acid, Heat*: In the **Heat** episode, Nosrat discusses how the heat of cooking can extract the depth of umami from ingredients like tomatoes, meat, and mushrooms. These rich, savory flavors provide a satisfying, nourishing experience and illustrate the transformative power of cooking as an alchemical process.

Heat doesn't just cook food—it unlocks hidden layers of flavor, textures, and aromas, deepening the sensory experience of a meal.

By coaxing out the umami through techniques like roasting, caramelizing, or slow simmering, heat enhances not only the taste but also the emotional satisfaction of eating. Nosrat reminds us that this process is not just about feeding the body but nourishing the soul, as it connects us to the elements, the ingredients, and the act of creation itself.

CONCLUSION

Allow cooking to become a mindful, sensory practice that invites you to fully engage with the present moment and the beauty of food and nourishment to feed the soul!

12
THE SIXTH SENSE: INTUITION

Each of us possess an inherent potential —an ability to assess the energies in our physical bodies, psyches, and beyond- a *sixth sense, or intuition* that helps us to do so.

In this chapter, we will explore intuition through the lenses of the physical anatomy associated, Chinese Medicine principles, Yogic philosophy, and Naturalist traditions, examining how these perspectives emphasize the importance of energetic awareness and balance.

By learning to recognize and trust our intuitive capabilities, we can deepen our connection to the wisdom within us, empowering ourselves to navigate health, healing, and life with greater clarity and ease.

The "sixth sense" or one's "intuition"- is a concept that transcends traditional, allopathic medical approaches and scientific explanations. Lets explore a few other thoughts and perspectives on the subject related to our discussion so far.

THE PINEAL GLAND, THE "SEAT OF INTUITION"

The pineal gland, often called the "seat of the soul" by philosopher René Descartes, has been revered for centuries as the gateway to higher consciousness and deep intuition. Situated at the geometric center of the brain, this small endocrine gland plays a crucial role in regulating sleep cycles, hormone production, and the body's alignment with natural rhythms.

However, beyond its physiological function, the pineal gland has long been associated with spiritual insight, mystical experiences, and heightened awareness. In many traditions, including Hinduism, Buddhism, and ancient Egyptian spirituality, this gland corresponds to the Ajna chakra (Third Eye), representing clarity, perception beyond the physical, and the ability to receive intuitive knowledge.

One of the most striking and enigmatic references to the pineal gland can be found in the Vatican, home to the largest pinecone sculpture in the world. This massive bronze Pigna (pinecone) statue, located in the Courtyard of the Belvedere, is an ancient relic from the Roman Pantheon, believed to have once functioned as a water feature near a temple dedicated to Isis, an Egyptian goddess associated with wisdom and the mystical arts. Today, it remains a powerful symbol within the heart of Catholicism.

The presence of such a large pinecone statue at the Vatican raises thought-provoking questions: Is this an acknowledgment of the power of the human mind to access higher states of being? Does it symbolize hidden esoteric knowledge within the church's teachings? While the Vatican does not openly discuss the pinecone's meaning, its inclusion in one of the most sacred sites of Christianity suggests a deeper symbolic, and perhaps even scientific, relevance to the mystery of human consciousness.

Whether viewed through the lens of religion, mysticism, or neuroscience, the pineal gland remains a fascinating bridge between the physical and metaphysical realms—a key to understanding both the nature of consciousness and our connection to the divine.

THE CRISTA GALLI

Ok, let's nerd out on some more anatomy together!

This is to me, one of the fascinating anatomical structures in the human body- a small bony ridge located in the ethmoid bone at the front of the skull, between the eyebrows.

Th Crista Galli where connections between the pineal gland and our perception of the divine merge. The name "Crista Galli" translates to "crest of the rooster" and has deep symbolic connotations across cultures, often linked to awakening, resurrection, and spiritual enlightenment.

This ridge serves as the attachment point for the falx cerebri, a dural membrane that separates the two cerebral hemispheres, acting as a stabilizing structure within the brain. The Crista Galli's position in the skull is directly aligned with the pineal gland, suggesting an energetic or structural connection between the physical and metaphysical realms of perception. It is also where the pituitary gland sits which is often referred to as the "master gland" because it plays a critical role in regulating the body's hormonal balance, growth, metabolism, and stress response.

In esoteric teachings and mystic traditions, the Crista Galli, Pituitary and the Pineal gland together create a powerful axis of spiritual insight. Some believe that activating the Third Eye through practices such as meditation, breath work, and visualization can stimulate both the pineal gland and the energetic field surrounding the Crista Galli, creating an internal bridge between higher states of consciousness and embodied awareness. This connection also aligns with the concept of the crown chakra (Sahasrara), which governs direct communion with divine intelligence.

Modern neuroscience is beginning to explore the role of the pineal gland in neuroplasticity, DMT production, and its potential influence on human perception and altered states of awareness.

Ancient wisdom, however, has long recognized its role in visionary experiences, inner guidance, and our ability to transcend ordinary consciousness. By activating the pineal gland through practices like yoga, yoga nidra, qigong, sound healing, and deep meditation, we can enhance our innate intuition, awaken dormant spiritual faculties, and cultivate a profound sense of interconnectedness with the universe.

THE POWER OF MEDICAL INTUITION

Medical intuition is the ability to perceive and understand the deeper, often unseen causes of imbalance in the body and mind relating to Health. It is an innate or learned sensitivity that allows us to detect shifts in energy, emotional patterns, and environmental influences that contribute to health imbalances or dysfunction. Rather than focusing solely on physical symptoms, ancient traditions like Chinese medicine, Yoga, and Naturalist healing recognize the body and mind as interconnected systems, deeply influenced by the flow of energy (Qi or Prana), our ability to tune into this wisdom and nature.

The intuitive sense often presents itself more obviously as a gut feeling, an inner nudge, or a sudden knowing—guiding us toward greater awareness and alignment. It can serve as an internal compass, helping us sense when something is off, foresee potential challenges, or recognize deeper truths about ourselves and others.

These flashes of insight, far from being mystical or rare, are a natural part of human perception and can be cultivated to enhance well-being and decision-making.

THE ENERGETIC BODY: UNDERSTANDING IMBALANCES IN CHINESE MEDICINE

In Traditional Chinese Medicine (TCM), health is understood as a dynamic flow of Qi (Chi, "chee"), the vital life force that moves through the body's energetic pathways, known as meridians. This flow governs not only physical functions but also emotional, mental, and spiritual well-being. When Qi circulates freely and in balance, the body thrives.

However, when Qi becomes stagnant, deficient, or excessive, imbalance arises, potentially leading to illness and dysfunction, as explored in previous chapters.

Intuition plays a key role in understanding energy imbalances within TCM. A refined awareness of Qi allows practitioners—especially those trained in Medical Qigong—to sense subtle shifts, blockages, and disruptions before they fully manifest as physical symptoms. Tools such as pulse diagnosis, tongue diagnosis, and visual observation help practitioners detect disharmony, but energetic sensitivity and intuitive awareness elevate the process, allowing for a more profound understanding of a person's overall health. This would then allow a Medical Qi gong practitioner to teach methods for resolution or help to resolve them directly.

For instance, Liver Qi stagnation is a TCM diagnoses we use-commonly associated with emotional stress, frustration, and unresolved anger. If this stagnation is not addressed, it may manifest physically as headaches, digestive disturbances, eye strain, or menstrual irregularities.

An intuitive practitioner, attuned to the body's energy, may detect these imbalances early and work to clear stagnation—offering solutions, relief and preventing deeper, more chronic issues from taking hold.

Both Chinese medicine and Yogic traditions recognize that true healing requires a holistic approach, addressing not just symptoms but the root cause of imbalance.

TCM works with meridians and Qi, while Yoga aligns with Chakras, Nadis, and Prana—yet both systems affirm that intuition is an essential tool for detecting energetic disturbances, guiding healing, and restoring harmony to body, mind, and spirit.

YOGIC PERSPECTIVE: THE CHAKRA SYSTEM AND ENERGY HEALING

The yogic tradition provides a profound framework for understanding the energetic body and its deep connection to health, intuition, and overall well-being.

At the core of this system is the belief that energy, or prana, flows through specific centers in the body known as Chakras (Sanskrit for "wheels"). These seven primary Chakras, running from the base of the spine to the crown of the head, influence our physical, emotional, mental, and spiritual states.

Each Chakra corresponds to a specific element, governing different aspects of our existence. The Root Chakra (Muladhara), for example, is linked to stability, survival, and grounding, while the Heart Chakra (Anahata) is associated with love, compassion, and emotional healing.

When a Chakra is blocked or imbalanced, it may manifest as emotional distress, mental fog, or physical ailments such as chronic pain, digestive issues, or fatigue.

The Ajna Chakra, or Third Eye Chakra, located between the eyebrows, is considered the center of intuition, insight, and higher perception. It is associated with light and governs our ability to see beyond the physical world, accessing deeper truths and inner guidance.

In yogic traditions, practices are taught for strengthening our ability to trust this Chakra for how to make aligned decisions and connect to higher consciousness. When this energy center is open and balanced, we experience clarity, deep knowing, and a strong sense of purpose. However, when blocked, it can lead to confusion, self-doubt, anxiety, and an inability to see the bigger picture.

Traditional Chinese Medicine (TCM) parallels this understanding, linking intuition to the Heart and Kidney energies, where wisdom is cultivated through stillness and deep listening.

Just as the Kidneys store essence (Jing) and provide the foundation for longevity, the Heart serves as the "empress/emperor," allowing us to process emotions and access inner wisdom.

To bring balance to the Chakras and energy systems, yogic practices such as pranayama (breath work), asana (postures), mantra chanting, and meditation are used as tools for self-awareness and energetic alignment. Practices such as Yoga Nidra, visualization, and alternate-nostril breathing (Nadi Shodhana) help activate the Ajna Chakra, strengthening the bridge between the logical mind and intuitive knowing.

Or as a physical example, lower back pain may indicate a blockage in the Root Chakra, while throat/neck tension or difficulty expressing oneself could be connected to the Throat Chakra (Vishuddhi).

A trained practitioner can often sense energy blockages in the Chakras, identifying emotional or spiritual imbalances before they manifest as physical discomfort or illness.

By tuning in to these subtle energy patterns, we can cultivate a deeper awareness of ourselves and others, supporting emotional release and energetic realignment.

Incorporating these ancient practices into daily life allows us to develop our intuition, refine our perception, and deepen our connection to both our inner world and the universe around us. Through the balance of body, breath, and awareness, we open ourselves to greater clarity, wisdom, and healing—unlocking the profound intelligence that resides within.

YOGIC PRACTICES TO ACTIVATE THE THIRD EYE & PITUITARY GLAND

To bring balance to the Chakras and energy systems, yogic practices such as pranayama (breath work), asana (postures), mantra chanting, and meditation are used as tools for self-awareness and energetic alignment.

Specific techniques that help to strengthen the inner vision include:

- **Shambhavi Mudra (Eyebrow Gazing):** A meditation practice where you gently focus the gaze upward toward the space between the eyebrows, stimulating the Ajna Chakra and pituitary gland.
- **Nadi Shodhana (Alternate Nostril Breathing):** This practice helps to balance the nervous system and harmonize the body's subtle energies, supporting the pituitary gland.
- **Khechari Mudra (Tongue Lock):** An advanced practice where the tongue is placed against the soft palate, believed to activate the pituitary and pineal glands, enhancing spiritual perception.

MEDICAL QIGONG: HARNESSING ENERGY FOR HEALING

Medical Qigong is a powerful, ancient practice rooted in Traditional Chinese Medicine (TCM) that focuses on cultivating, balancing, and directing Qi (vital energy) to promote healing and overall well-being. As one of the foundational branches of TCM—alongside acupuncture, herbal medicine, and bodywork—Medical Qigong integrates movement, breath work, visualization, and energetic awareness to support the body's natural healing processes.

Unlike conventional exercise, Medical Qigong works directly with the meridian system and energy field, helping to remove stagnation, clear blockages, and restore harmony to the organs and subtle body. It is often used to boost immunity, relieve stress, support emotional balance, and aid recovery from illness or injury by guiding Qi through intentional movement and focused intention.

Practicing Medical Qigong involves a combination of gentle postures (similar to yoga but unique to Qigong), controlled breathing techniques, and meditative focus to regulate energy flow. Some exercises are prescriptive, targeting specific organ imbalances, while others are designed to increase vitality and longevity.

This practice can be done as a self-healing method or facilitated by a trained Qigong practitioner to assist in directing Qi for deeper energetic restoration.

At its core, Medical Qigong empowers individuals to become active participants in their own healing or the healing of others, fostering a profound connection between body, mind, and spirit.

By working in harmony with the rhythms of nature and the internal wisdom of the body, this practice and study offer a deeply transformative approach to health, balance, and holistic well-being.

THE NATURALIST PERSPECTIVE: TUNING INTO THE BODY AND THE RHYTHMS OF NATURE

From a naturalist perspective, intuition is not a mystical force but an innate cognitive ability—a skill honed through experience, pattern recognition, and deep connection with the natural world. Often described as a "gut feeling," intuition emerges from the brain's complex processing of sensory input, past experiences, and environmental cues, allowing for quick, instinctive decision-making without conscious reasoning. This view emphasizes that intuition is a natural phenomenon shaped by our direct interactions with the world around us rather than something supernatural.

In this context, intuition is about listening—both to the body and to nature. Human beings are not separate from the ecosystems they inhabit; rather, we are intricately woven into the cycles of the seasons, the phases of the moon, and the ever-changing natural landscape. When we fall out of sync with these rhythms, whether through overwork, poor diet, lack of movement, or excessive indoor living, our bodies send signals—fatigue, digestive issues, shifts in appetite, disturbed sleep, or emotional imbalances—indicating a need for realignment with nature.

A naturalist approach to healing focuses on restoring balance through nature's wisdom, using the body's own intuitive healing mechanisms, whole foods, herbal medicine, movement, and time spent in natural environments to support overall well-being.

Intuition, in this sense, is the ability to recognize what the body truly needs at any given time—whether it's fresh air after long periods indoors, nutrient-dense whole foods to counteract processed meals, or deep rest after prolonged exertion.

If for example, you are feeling drained after days of artificial lighting and screen exposure, this naturally signals the need for time outdoors in natural sunlight to restore your energy.

A craving for bitter greens or mineral-rich broths could indicate a need for digestive support or mineral replenishment. Instead of seeing illness simply as a problem to be fixed, a naturalist approach views it as a message—a sign that something in one's life is out of harmony and needs attention.

By tuning into these subtle cues and spending intentional time in nature without distractions, we strengthen our connection to the body's innate intelligence.

Intuitively choosing healing foods, herbal remedies, or self-care practices based on the body's needs fosters deep trust in both nature and oneself, guiding us toward greater health, balance and overall vitality.

INTUITION AS A BRIDGE BETWEEN MIND, BODY, AND SPIRIT

Ultimately, intuition serves as a bridge between the physical body and the energetic, emotional, and spiritual dimensions of health. It allows us to access deeper levels of awareness, uncovering the root causes of illness and imbalance that may not be immediately visible in the physical body.

By understanding the subtle energies that govern our health, we can begin to address not only the symptoms but also the underlying emotional and spiritual factors that contribute to disease.

Practical ways to enhance your Intuition:

1. **Cultivate Mindful Awareness:** Through practices like meditation, yoga, or breath work, you can develop a heightened awareness of your body and emotions. Pay attention to sensations, thoughts, and feelings without judgment and tune into the subtle energies that influence your health and cycles in life.
2. **Develop an Intuitive Connection with Nature**: Spend time in natural environments—whether in the forest, by the ocean, or in a garden. Let your gaze soften as you listen to the elements and signs around you. Nature provides the perfect setting to reconnect with your body's natural rhythms and attune to the ever present energetic forces.
3. **Listen to Your Body**: Learn to listen to your body's signals, including hunger, fatigue, pain, and mood changes. These are messages that can offer insight into underlying imbalances. In Chinese medicine, a feeling of cold in the body may indicate a deficiency of Yang, while persistent fatigue could point to a deficiency in Qi for example. Choose nutrition and practices that bring more of what is needed.
4. **Seek Balance in All Areas of Life:** True healing requires balance in all aspects of life—diet, movement, relationships, and emotional health. Not always easy, AND, doesn't have to be perfect! By attuning to your body's needs and cultivating balance, you can help to prevent illness before it manifests physically.

CONCLUSION: THE HEALING POTENTIAL OF INTUITION

Each of us has the capacity to tap into deeper insights about our health, accessing the wisdom of the body, mind, and spirit through the sense of Intuition. By becoming more attuned to our physical and energetic states, we can identify and address the underlying causes of imbalance and illness.

Utilizing this sense of intuition offers a profound pathway to restoring harmony and achieving true wellness. With practice and awareness, we can unlock our inner healing potential and live in alignment with the rhythms of life, the earth, and the universe.

PART III
THE WISDOM OF THE SEASONS

In Part three, we will focus on helpful TCM, Yoga, Qigong, Nutrition, Aromatherapy and Meditations specifically designed to support and inspire your optimal health and vitality year round.

The changing of the seasons reflects the natural cycles of life—birth, growth, transformation, rest, and renewal. Each season carries a distinct energy that influences our health, emotions, and spiritual state.

- **Spring | The Wood Element:** A season of renewal and growth
- **Summer | The Fire Element:** A season of radiance and expansion
- **Late Summer | The Earth Element:** A season of nurturing and harvest
- **Autumn | The Metal Element:** A season of release and transformation
- **Winter | The Water Element:** A season of stillness and reflection

13
SPRING- REBIRTH, RENEWAL AND GROWTH

<u>The Dance of Awakening</u>

Tender buds stretch toward the sky,
Spring's breath whispers, soft and wild.
A canvas of green in vibrant hue,
Awakens the earth with life anew.
Roots grow deep, yet branches rise,
Reaching upward, strong and spry.
The Wood element's dance unfolds,
Energy surging, fresh and bold.
Through twists and bends, we find release,
Flowing like rivers, embracing peace.
Stretching open, swaying free,
the trees yet strong as ever they be.
With eyes wide open, we behold,
The blessings of Spring, both bright and yet untold.
A season of growth, of movement and grace,
Inviting renewal in nature's embrace.

—Erika Hawley

SPRING - A SEASON OF RENEWAL AND GROWTH

Spring is a time filled with possibility—both in the natural world and within ourselves. Just as the earth awakens, and new buds blossom, so too do our potential for new beginnings, fresh ideas, and new ways of being.

In Chinese medicine, spring is associated with the Wood element, which represents growth, vitality, and the energy of new beginnings. During this season, we are invited to shed the heaviness of winter and reemerge with a renewed sense of purpose and vitality.

Just as the earth begins to awaken from its cold dormancy, so too can we engage our senses and align our mind and body with the energy of renewal and growth. By participating in simple, mindful exercises, we can deepen our connection to the season and embrace its transformative potential.

The Wood element in Chinese medicine is linked to the Liver (Yin organ) and the Gallbladder (Yang organ). Together, these organs help regulate the smooth flow of energy (Qi) and facilitate the body's ability to grow, expand, and renew itself. Just as the first shoots of grass and tender leaves push through the soil after winter's dormancy, so can we tap into our inner potential for growth and expansion during spring.

Associations with Spring according to TCM:

Organs: Liver (Yin) and Gallbladder (Yang)
Sense Organ: Eyes
Tissues: Tendons and ligaments
Emotion: Anger (imbalanced), Kindness/Compassion (balanced)
Color: Green
Taste: Sour
Smell: Rancid
Energy: Renewal, growth, and expansion; the time to plant seeds, both literally and metaphorically.

Seasonal Focus: Detoxification and flow. The Liver's role is to ensure the smooth flow of Qi and emotions, as well as help with planning and decision-making.

WOOD ELEMENT AND THE EYES

The wood element is deeply connected to the sense of sight, as the Liver is believed to "open to the eyes" in TCM. As we step into the vitality of spring, we are invited to sharpen our vision—both physically and metaphorically. This is a time to clear the fog from our minds, set intentions, and see the world with renewed clarity. Practices such as eye exercises, spending time outdoors in fresh green spaces, and mindful movement like yoga and Qigong help harmonize the Wood element, supporting both our inner and outer vision as we step into the expansive energy of spring.

SPRING NOURISHMENT: A TIME FOR FRESH, LIGHT FOODS

Spring is the perfect time to lighten up your diet, embracing fresh and seasonal produce. This supports detoxification, boosts immunity, and provides essential nutrients for vitality and liver health.

Spring foods—leafy greens, sprouts, and fresh fruits like strawberries and green apples—are packed with antioxidants, fiber, vitamins, and minerals that nourish the body and mind.

Foods that are light, fresh, slightly sour, and fiber-rich support detoxification, energy flow, and renewal.

1. **Leafy Greens & Detoxifying Vegetables** *(Aid digestion & Liver detoxification)*

- Spinach, kale, bok choy, dandelion greens, watercress, mustard greens, parsley, cilantro
- Asparagus, celery, scallions, leeks, radishes, Brussels sprouts

2. Sour & Cleansing Fruits *(Aid Liver detoxification)*

- Lemon, lime, grapefruit, green apples, cherries, plums
- Berries (strawberries, blueberries, raspberries, mulberries)

3. Fermented & Probiotic Foods *(Aid digestion & Liver detoxification)*

- Sauerkraut, kimchi, miso, apple cider vinegar, kombucha, pickled vegetables

4. Whole Grains & Fiber-Rich Foods *(Support digestion & balance energy levels)*

- Quinoa, barley, brown rice, millet, oats

5. Legumes & Nuts *(Gentle cleansing & nourishment)*

- Mung beans, lentils, adzuki beans, chickpeas
- Pumpkin seeds, sunflower seeds, walnuts, flaxseeds

6. Herbs & Spices for Liver Support *(Improve circulation & aid digestion)*

- Ginger, turmeric, peppermint, milk thistle, dandelion root, hawthorn berry, basil

7. Light Proteins & Healthy Fats *(Reduce Liver burden & provide nourishment)*

- Free-range chicken, duck, white fish, eggs, tofu (moderation)
- Avocados, olive oil, sesame oil

8. Spring Teas & Hydrating Drinks *(Detoxifying & cooling for the Liver)*

- Green tea, dandelion tea, lemon water, chrysanthemum tea, peppermint tea

DIETARY TIPS FOR SPRING:

1. **Embrace Fresh, Seasonal Produce:** Focus on leafy greens, sprouts, asparagus, peas, radishes, and strawberries. These foods support detoxification, boost immunity, and promote liver health.
2. **Lighten Up Your Diet:** Transition to lighter, easier-to-digest foods like salads, steamed vegetables, and lighter proteins such as fish or tofu. Reduce heavy meats and processed foods.
3. **Hydrate with Fresh Infusions:** Add slices of citrus, cucumber, or mint to your water for a refreshing boost of vitamins and hydration.
4. **Incorporate Bitter and Pungent Foods:** Include dandelion greens, arugula, and ginger, which help stimulate digestion and promote energy flow.
5. **Focus on Green Juices and Smoothies:** These nutrient-dense beverages can support detoxification and provide essential vitamins and minerals for vitality.

Spring is a time to align your body and mind with the rhythms of nature, embracing the season of growth, expansion, and new beginnings. By engaging with the world around you and nourishing yourself from the inside out, you can fully harness the energy of spring to transform and renew your life.

HARMONIZING THE WOOD ELEMENT: YOGA, PRANAYAMA, MEDITATION AND AROMATHERAPY FOR SPRING

Incorporating specific yoga poses into your practice can help stimulate and harmonize the Liver and Gallbladder meridians, promoting flexibility, detoxification, emotional balance, and physical strength.

Tree Pose (Vrksasana)

How to Practice:

1. Stand tall with feet hip-width apart.
2. Shift your weight onto one foot, rooting it firmly into the ground.
3. Bring the sole of the opposite foot to the inner thigh or calf (avoid placing it on the knee).
4. Press hands together at heart center or extend arms overhead like branches.
5. Maintain a steady gaze (Drishti) to enhance balance.
6. Hold for 5–10 breaths, then switch sides.

Benefits:

- Strengthens the legs, ankles, and core.
- Enhances balance and concentration.
- Encourages grounding while embracing expansion, reflecting the energy of Spring and the Wood element.
- Stimulates the Liver meridian, promoting smooth Qi flow and emotional resilience.

Warrior II (Virabhadrasana II)

How to Practice:

1. Step feet wide apart, turning one foot out 90 degrees and the back foot slightly in.
2. Bend the front knee to stack over the ankle, keeping the back leg strong and engaged.
3. Extend arms parallel to the floor, gazing over the front fingertips.

4. Hold for 5–10 breaths, feeling strong and stable, then switch sides.

Benefits:

- Builds endurance and strengthens the lower body.
- Expands the chest and hips, enhancing flexibility.
- Activates the Liver and Gallbladder meridians, moving stagnant energy.
- Fosters inner strength, courage, and clarity—key attributes of Spring's renewing energy.

<u>Twisted Chair Pose (Parivrtta Utkatasana)</u>

How to Practice:

1. Stand with feet together and bend the knees, lowering the hips as if sitting in a chair.
2. Bring hands to heart center and twist the torso, hooking one elbow outside the opposite knee.
3. Press palms together, lengthening through the spine as you deepen the twist.
4. Hold for 5–7 breaths, then switch sides.

Benefits:

- Stimulates digestion, aiding the Liver and Gallbladder meridians in their detoxification process.
- Strengthens the legs and core while increasing spinal mobility.
- Encourages the release of emotional stagnation and promotes mental clarity.
- Supports Spring's energy of renewal by wringing out the old to make space for the new to enter.

<u>Fish Pose (Matsyasana)</u>

How to Practice:

1. Lie on your back with legs extended.
2. Place hands under hips, pressing elbows into the mat.
3. Lift the chest, arching the back and tilting the head back, either resting on the crown of the head or keeping it slightly lifted.
4. Hold for 5–10 breaths, breathing deeply into the chest.

Benefits:

- Opens the chest, throat, and abdomen, encouraging emotional release.
- Stimulates the Liver meridian, particularly around the rib cage and diaphragm, where frustration and tension can accumulate.
- Improves lung capacity and enhances circulation.
- Encourages emotional balance and Spring's energy of growth and expansion.

Cat-Cow (Marjaryasana) with Side-to-Side Tail Wags

How to Practice:

1. Begin in a tabletop position with wrists under shoulders and knees under hips.
2. Inhale, lift the tailbone and heart for Cow Pose.
3. Exhale, round the spine and tuck the chin for Cat Pose.
4. Repeat for several breaths, moving fluidly.
5. To add tail wags, keep the spine neutral and gently sway hips toward one side while turning your head to look back at your feet.
6. Switch sides, moving rhythmically for 6–8 breaths.

Benefits:

- Awakens the spine and stimulates the Liver and Gallbladder meridians, which govern flexibility.
- Promotes circulation and detoxification, supporting the Wood element.
- Enhances spinal mobility and emotional fluidity, helping to release stagnation.
- Encourages a sense of playfulness and movement, mirroring the growth and expansion of Spring.

PRANAYAMA (BREATHING TECHNIQUES) FOR SPRING

Incorporating mindful breathing techniques into your practice can help enhance the flow of Qi, promote clarity, and release stagnant energy. Two powerful breathing techniques that support the Wood element and balance the Liver and Gallbladder meridians are:

Nadi Shodhana (Alternate Nostril Breathing)

Balances Energy, Calms the Mind, and Supports Liver Meridian Function

How to Practice:

1. Sit comfortably with your spine upright and shoulders relaxed.
2. Place your left hand on your knee, palm facing up in a relaxed position.
3. Use Nasagra Mudra with your right hand (Place the index and middle fingers on the eyebrow center. Relax your hand. Use your right thumb to close your right nostril. Use your ring finger to close your left nostril)
4. Close your right nostril with your thumb.
5. Inhale deeply through the left nostril, filling your lungs completely.
6. Close the left nostril with your ring finger, release your thumb, and exhale through the right nostril.
7. Inhale through the right nostril, then close it and exhale through the left.

8. Continue alternating for 5-10 rounds, maintaining a smooth, steady rhythm.

Benefits:

- Clears energetic blockages in the Liver meridian, helping to ease emotional stagnation, frustration, or irritability.
- Balances the right and left hemispheres of the brain, improving focus, clarity, and emotional regulation.
- Soothes the nervous system, reducing anxiety and stress often heightened in the transition into spring.
- Supports the respiratory system by improving oxygen intake and detoxification.

Viloma Pranayama (Three-Part Breath to Awaken the Lungs)

Expands Lung Capacity, Enhances Circulation, and Encourages Flexibility

How to Practice:

1. Sit in a comfortable position with your spine elongated or lie down in Savasana.
2. Place one hand on your abdomen and the other on your chest to feel the breath's movement.
3. Begin by inhaling in three equal parts, pausing slightly between each inhale (for example: inhale 1/3 → pause → inhale 2/3 → pause → inhale full).
4. Exhale smoothly in one continuous breath, allowing the body to relax.
5. Alternatively, practice with segmented exhalation instead: take one full breath in, then release in three gentle steps, pausing briefly between each exhale.
6. Continue for 5-8 minutes, focusing on expanding and releasing tension in the lungs and diaphragm.

Benefits:

- Encourages slow, deep breathing, activating the parasympathetic nervous system and reducing stress.
- Improves lung capacity, flexibility, and oxygenation, which supports overall vitality and detoxification.
- Gently massages the diaphragm and Liver area, assisting in the smooth flow of Qi and blood circulation.
- Enhances patience and emotional resilience, mirroring the steady, organic growth of spring.
- By incorporating these two pranayama practices into your spring routine, you can cultivate balance, adaptability, and a deeper connection to your breath—supporting both physical and emotional well-being during this season of renewal.

MEDITATIONS FOR SPRING: CULTIVATING HARMONY AND EMOTIONAL BALANCE

Mindfulness Meditation

Cultivates Emotional Clarity, Reduces Stress, and Supports Liver Meridian Balance

How to Practice:

1. Find a comfortable seated position with your spine straight and shoulders relaxed. You may also lie down if that feels better.
2. Close your eyes or soften your gaze and take a few deep breaths to settle into the moment.
3. Bring your attention to your breath, observing its natural rhythm without trying to control it.
4. As thoughts, emotions, or sensations arise, acknowledge them without attachment—like clouds passing in the sky.
5. If your mind wanders, gently return your focus to your breath or a chosen anchor, such as bodily sensations or sounds around you.
6. Continue for 5-10 minutes or longer, allowing yourself to

fully experience the present moment with openness and curiosity.

Benefits:

- Helps release stagnant emotions stored in the Liver meridian, such as frustration, irritability, or resentment.
- Encourages emotional regulation, reducing reactivity and improving patience.
- Enhances mental clarity and awareness, helping you respond rather than react to challenges.
- Supports overall nervous system balance, fostering a sense of calm and inner stability.

Loving-Kindness Meditation (Metta)

Cultivates Compassion, Emotional Healing, and Balance in the Liver and Gallbladder Meridians

How to Practice:

1. Sit comfortably with your hands resting on your lap or over your heart.
2. Close your eyes and take a few deep breaths, softening your body and mind.
3. Silently repeat phrases such as: "May I be happy. May I be healthy. May I be free from suffering. May I live with ease."
4. After a few minutes, extend these wishes to someone you love: "May you be happy. May you be healthy. May you be free from suffering. May you live with ease."
5. Next, extend kindness to a neutral person (someone you feel indifferent toward) and then to someone you may have difficulties with.
6. Finally, radiate this loving energy to all beings: "May all beings be happy. May all beings be healthy. May all beings be free from suffering."

7. Sit in this warmth of compassion for a few minutes before gently bringing your awareness back to the present moment.

Benefits:

- Softens emotional imbalances linked to the Liver and Gallbladder, such as resentment and suppressed anger.
- Encourages heart-centered awareness, increasing feelings of love, gratitude, and connection.
- Helps release emotional blockages that can manifest as tension or stagnation in the body.
- Strengthens emotional resilience and promotes a sense of peace and well-being.

Both mindfulness and loving-kindness meditation offer profound healing benefits, allowing you to navigate life's transitions with greater ease, patience, and openness—just as spring invites new beginnings and fresh possibilities.

QI GONG FOR SPRING: FOCUSING ON THE LIVER MERIDIAN AND EYES

Qi gong is an ancient Chinese practice that combines movement, breath, and meditation to cultivate and balance Qi throughout the body.

"Liver Detox Flow" (Wood Element – Liver & Gallbladder)

Purpose: This practice supports the Liver and Gallbladder meridians, clearing out stagnation and encouraging the free flow of Qi (life force energy).

How to Practice:

1. Stand Tall in Wuji Posture – Feet hip-width apart, knees slightly bent, arms relaxed.

2. Inhale & Reach Up – Slowly raise your arms overhead, fingers spread wide like branches growing toward the sky. Open Eyes wide and look around!
3. Exhale & Twist – Gently twist your torso to the left, looking over your left shoulder, arms sweeping down like a willow tree bending in the wind.
4. Inhale & Return to Center – Bring your arms back overhead.
5. Exhale & Twist to the Right – Flow into the twist on the other side.
6. Repeat for 6–10 rounds, moving fluidly with your breath and allowing your body to follow your gaze.
7. Focus on deep, cleansing breaths, releasing stored emotions and toxins.

SENSORY ACTIVITIES

Sound: Connect with Nature's Symphony

Outdoor Yoga: Take your yoga practice or meditation outdoors, where the sounds of nature—birds chirping, leaves rustling in the wind, and the gentle hum of the earth—become your soundtrack. Practicing in an outdoor setting allows you to align with the natural world's rhythm, helping you feel grounded and present in the moment. The soothing sounds of spring not only calm the nervous system but also support a deeper sense of connection to the earth's restorative energy.

Deep Listening Meditation: Spend time outside in nature and practice deep listening. Focus on individual sounds—the chirp of a bird, the rustle of wind, the distant hum of a stream. Allow each sound to arise and fade away without judgment, just observing. This practice enhances mindfulness and creates space for a deeper understanding of the subtle energies in the environment around you.

Taste: Savor the Fresh Flavors of Spring

Farmer's Market Visit: Embrace the flavors of the season by visiting a local farmer's market. Spring is a time when the earth's abundance presents itself in vibrant, fresh produce—think juicy strawberries, crisp asparagus, and tender leafy greens. Savor each bite, noticing the texture, sweetness, and freshness. These flavors not only nourish the body but also bring a deeper appreciation for the seasonal cycle and the nourishment the earth provides.

Mindful Eating: In addition to exploring fresh produce, practice mindful eating by fully engaging your senses. Savor each bite slowly, paying attention to the textures, flavors, and sensations of the food in your mouth. By eating mindfully, you align your body with the earth's cycles and cultivate a deeper connection to both your body and the planet.

Smell: Awaken the Senses with Aromatherapy and Nature

Flower Garden Tour: Visit a botanical garden or flower farm to indulge your sense of smell with the rich, fragrant aromas of spring blooms. Roses, lilacs, jasmine, and tulips offer a symphony of scents that awaken the spirit and refresh the mind. The act of inhaling the natural scents of flowers can help clear mental fog, calm the nerves, and lift your mood.

Aromatherapy Blends: Create a springtime aromatherapy blend (we have one in the DIY section for you!) using essential oils like lavender, peppermint, and citrus. Diffuse this blend throughout your home or apply it to your wrists or temples to immerse yourself in the refreshing and rejuvenating qualities of these natural scents. Aromatherapy can evoke powerful emotional responses, grounding and uplifting you as you embrace the energy of spring.

Touch: Ground Yourself in the Earth

Picnic on the Grass: Feel the soft, green grass beneath your hands and feet as you enjoy a picnic outdoors. The tactile experience of being in direct contact with the earth helps you feel grounded and connected to nature. Soak in the warmth of the sun on your skin, breathing in the fresh air and feeling the earth's nurturing energy. This simple yet profound practice can help restore balance and invigorate your body and mind.

Self-Massage with Scented Oils: After a day spent outdoors, practice self-massage using essential oils or nourishing lotions. Pay special attention to areas that feel tense or tired, such as the shoulders, neck, or feet. By massaging these areas with natural oils, you not only soothe physical tension but also provide your body with a sensory experience that promotes relaxation, rejuvenation and grounding.

Sight: Invigorate the Eyes with Spring's Beauty

Mindful Nature Walks: Take a mindful walk through a park or forest, focusing on the sights of spring—the vibrant colors of blooming flowers, the new buds on trees, and the fresh greenery that blankets the landscape. Spring's colors—the soft pastels of flowers, the vibrant greens of the grass—can help to lift your spirit and rejuvenate your senses. Notice how the light changes throughout the day and how the colors shift as the season progresses.

Eye Yoga: Just as the body benefits from physical exercise, the eyes also need care and attention. Practice eye yoga to strengthen and relax your eye muscles. Simple exercises like palming (rubbing your palms together and gently cupping your eyes- refer to the section on Sight for more specific practices), blinking, and eye rotations can improve focus and reduce eye strain. These exercises are particularly beneficial as the bright, vibrant sights of spring awaken your eyes and your senses- especially bright green colors!

AROMATHERAPY FOR SPRING: SUPPORTING THE WOOD ELEMENT

Below are some essential oils that can support you during the spring season:

1. Lavender

Lavender is a calming oil that promotes **relaxation** and **balance**, helping ease the tensions and emotional blockages associated with the Liver. Its soothing properties can be especially helpful when navigating the transition into spring.

2. Lemon

Lemon's bright, citrusy aroma is **energizing** and **uplifting**, helping to invigorate the senses and clear stagnant energy. Lemon oil supports the Liver's detoxifying function and promotes mental clarity.

3. Peppermint

Peppermint oil has a refreshing, **cooling** scent that stimulates the mind and clears mental fog. It enhances focus, refreshes the spirit, and supports clarity of thought—ideal for spring's energy of renewal.

4. Geranium

Geranium offers a **balancing** and **harmonizing** effect, helping to uplift the mood and promote emotional equilibrium. It is especially helpful for the Liver, as it supports the release of repressed emotions like frustration and anger.

5. Grapefruit

Grapefruit oil is an energizing oil that helps **boost energy** and **invigorate** the spirit. Its refreshing scent uplifts the mood and supports a positive outlook during the transition from winter to spring.

6. Ylang Ylang

Ylang Ylang is a calming and uplifting oil known for its ability to reduce **stress** and **enhance relaxation.** It helps promote emotional balance and is especially helpful in releasing feelings of anger or tension stored in the Liver.

7. Eucalyptus

Eucalyptus oil provides a **refreshing** and **clearing** scent that supports respiratory health and offers mental clarity. It helps clear emotional blockages and promote physical vitality.

8. Rosemary

Rosemary is a stimulating herbaceous oil that improves **focus,**

mental clarity, and **alertness**. It is perfect for clearing stagnant energy and stimulating the flow of Qi in the Liver meridian.

9. Bergamot

Bergamot has an uplifting and citrusy aroma that helps **reduce stress** and **promote emotional balance**, making it ideal for the Liver. It encourages openness, relaxation, and emotional well-being.

10. Clary Sage

Clary Sage oil helps promote **relaxation**, **balance hormones**, and support emotional well-being. It is particularly helpful during seasonal transitions, offering comfort and stability.

USING ESSENTIAL OILS SAFELY

As with all essential oils, be sure to follow proper dilution and usage guidelines. When using citrus oils, such as Lemon and Bergamot, be cautious of photo sensitivity. Always consult a qualified aromatherapist or healthcare professional for personalized guidance, especially if you have specific health concerns. *Refer to Part 3: Chapter 8- Smell, for more information on the Safe usage of essential oils.

CONCLUSION

As we move into spring and embrace the energy of the Wood element, let these practices—yoga, pranayama, meditation, Qi gong, and aromatherapy—be your guide to balancing the Liver and Gallbladder meridians and supporting your physical, emotional, and energetic health. Listen to your body, honor your emotions, and allow the flow of life to unfold with ease, vitality, and clarity. The energy of spring is one of renewal, growth, and potential, and by nurturing these practices, you can align yourself.

14
SUMMER-RADIANCE AND EXPANSION

Flames of Passion

In flames of passion, a truth ignites,
Illuminating the path to what is right.
Fire flickers, yearning, bold—
Stoke its glow, let love unfold.
Move with purpose, let it show,
Let the whole world truly know—
The strength within, the flame inside,
A soul unshaken, open wide.
For truth endures beyond all time,
Residing in your heart and mind.
Let it burn, let it shine—
A light that leads, both yours and mine.

—Erika Hawley

SUMMER: A SEASON OF EXPANSION, WARMTH, AND VIBRANCY

Summer is a time of expansion, joy, and connection, and it corresponds with the Fire element in Chinese Medicine. When the world around us is in full bloom, and our bodies and spirits are invited to engage in the richness of life and expand as well.

Just as the days lengthen and the sun's warmth intensifies, our inner energy awakens, inviting us to express ourselves more fully, connect with others, and celebrate life.

The Fire element is associated with the Heart (Yin organ) and Small Intestine (Yang organ). Together, these organs regulate our vitality, emotion, and digestive health. Summer is a season to nurture our hearts, build community, and honor our creative and expressive energies.

<u>Associations with Summer according to TCM:</u>

- **Organs:** Heart (Yin) and Small Intestine (Yang)
- **Sense Organ:** Tongue
- **Tissues:** Blood vessels
- **Emotion:** Joy (balanced), Over excitement/Agitation (imbalanced)
- **Color:** Red
- **Taste:** Bitter
- **Smell:** Scorched
- **Energy:** Fullness, passion, and outward expression; the time of peak energy and celebration.
- **Seasonal Focus:** Cultivating joy, connection, and overall circulation. Supports the Heart's role in governing the mind (Shen) and emotional well-being.

****Secondary Organs for Summer and all Seasons:**

- **Pericardium (Yin):** Also known as the Heart Protector, governs emotional expression and balances heart energy.
- **Triple Burner/San Jiao (Yang):** Responsible for regulating energy flow and balancing body temperature across the upper, middle, and lower parts of the body.

Notes:

- Each season is linked to an element in the Five Element Theory (Wood, Fire, Earth, Metal, Water).
- The secondary Fire meridians (Pericardium and Triple Burner) are not tied to a specific season but function to maintain balance and harmony throughout all seasons.

FIRE ELEMENT AND THE TONGUE: THE SENSORY CONNECTION

In summer, the tongue plays a vital role in experiencing the Fire element through taste. As the Fire element governs the sense of taste, our taste buds come alive with the abundance of fresh fruits, vegetables, and summer delicacies. This is the time to indulge in the bittersweet tastes of summer as the tongue becomes particularly attuned to these flavors.

SUMMER NUTRITIONAL RECOMMENDATIONS

To maintain balance and health during the summer months, it is essential to support the Fire element with cooling, hydrating, and light foods. Focus on fresh, seasonal produce that nourishes the body without overwhelming it with heaviness or excess heat.

Foods that are cooling, hydrating, bitter, and vibrant help regulate heat, support circulation, and maintain balance.

1. **Hydrating Fruits & Vegetables** *(Cool the body & prevent dehydration)*

- Watermelon, cantaloupe, honeydew, cucumber

- Tomatoes, zucchini, lettuce, celery, radishes
- Bell peppers, bitter melon, summer squash

2. Cooling & Bitter Greens *(Promote circulation & Heart balance)*

- Romaine lettuce, arugula, endive, dandelion greens, chicory
- Spinach, kale, Swiss chard

3. Light & Easy-to-Digest Whole Grains *(Sustain energy without overheating the body)*

•Quinoa, amaranth, barley, millet, brown rice

4. Lean Proteins & Plant-Based Alternatives *(Support muscle function & digestion in hot weather)*

•Fish (salmon, cod, trout), free-range chicken, tofu, eggs

•Mung beans, chickpeas, lentils

5. Healthy Fats & Cooling Oils *(Nourish the body without heaviness)*

•Avocado, coconut oil, flaxseeds, sesame oil, extra virgin olive oil

6. Fermented & Probiotic-Rich Foods *(Aid digestion & balance internal heat)*

•Miso, kimchi, sauerkraut, yogurt, pickled vegetables

7. Cooling & Bitter Herbs *(Reduce internal heat & promote detoxification)*

•Mint, cilantro, basil, dill, parsley, dandelion root

•Chrysanthemum, hibiscus, red clover

8. Hydrating Drinks & Herbal Teas *(Support digestion & reduce summer heat)*

•Lemon water, coconut water, green tea, hibiscus tea

•Mint, chrysanthemum, mung bean and barley tea

SUMMER EATING TIPS:

1. **Favor cooling, water-rich foods** to stay hydrated and prevent heat accumulation.
2. **Incorporate bitter and lightly pungent flavors** (arugula, dandelion greens, radishes) to balance the Fire element.
3. **Avoid excessive spicy, fried, and greasy foods**, as they create excess heat and sluggish digestion.
4. **Eat smaller, more frequent meals** to avoid overburdening digestion in hot weather.
5. **Embrace fresh seasonal produce:** Focus on the vibrant, nutrient-dense foods that are abundant during summer. These not only nourish the body but also support detoxification and energy levels.

EMBRACING THE FIRE ELEMENT: YOGA, PRANAYAMA, MEDITATION AND AROMATHERAPY FOR SUMMER

Yoga poses in the summer season focus on heart-opening asanas, energizing poses, and poses that stimulate both emotional and physical vitality.

Here are some key poses to incorporate into your practice:

<u>Sun Salutations (Surya Namaskar)</u>

How to Practice:

1. Begin standing with a tall spine in Prayer Pose (Pranamasana) with hands at the heart center.
2. Inhale, reach arms overhead into Raised arms pose (Hasta uttanasana).
3. Exhale, fold forward into Hand to Foot pose (Padahastasana).
4. Inhale, place hands beside your left foot and step back with the right foot. Keep the front knee bent and right toes on the

floor. Extend through the right leg and lift up through the spine (Ashwa Sanchalanasana).

5. Exhale, step left foot back into Mountain pose(Parvatasana-also reffered to as Downward Facing-Dog-Adho Mukha Svanasana)
6. Lower to Knees chest and chin into Eight point salute (Ashtanga Namaskara)
7. Inhale, lift into Cobra Pose (Bhujangasana).
8. Exhale, push back into Mountain Pose (Downward Facing Dog)
9. Inhale, step forward with the left foot into (ashwa sanchalasana), lift through the crown of the head
10. Exhale, step feet together and exhale back into Hand to Foot pose or forward fold (Padahastasana)
11. Inhale, rise to stand, reach arms overhead in Raised arms Pose (Hasta Uttanasana)
12. Then exhale back to Standing Prayer pose (Pranamasana)

**This completes half of one round. Begin the second half by stepping back with the left foot this time, to balance and strengthen both sides of the body. Practice up to 10 rounds- first 3 rounds slowly, 3 rounds more vigorously and the last 3 rounds slowly.

Benefits:

- Stimulates circulation and warms the body, making it an excellent morning practice.
- Activates the Solar Plexus, Heart, and Small Intestine meridians, bringing balance to summer's fiery energy.
- Improves flexibility, strengthens muscles, and boosts overall vitality.

<u>Precautions for Practicing Surya Namaskar (Sun Salutations)</u>**

Surya Namaskar is a dynamic sequence that offers numerous benefits, including improved flexibility, strength, circulation, and mental clarity. However, like any physical practice, it should be approached with awareness and caution. Below are key precautions to keep in mind before incorporating Surya Namaskar into your routine.

1. Practice on an Empty Stomach

- Ideally, perform Surya Namaskar in the morning before eating or at least 2-3 hours after a meal to avoid discomfort during the practice.

2. Warm-Up if Needed

- If you have stiff joints or muscles, perform gentle stretches or warm-up movements before beginning the sequence to prevent strain or injury.

3. Respect Your Body's Limits

- Do not force yourself into deep stretches, backbends, or forward folds.
- Modify poses as needed, especially if you have limited flexibility, injuries, or chronic conditions.

4. Avoid Holding the Breath

- Breath control is essential in Surya Namaskar. Maintain smooth, continuous breathing synchronized with each movement. Holding the breath can cause strain and dizziness.

5. Precautions for Specific Health Conditions

- **High Blood Pressure & Heart Conditions** – Avoid fast-paced sequences, excessive backbends, or prolonged breath retention. Practice slowly and mindfully.
- **Back Issues & Herniated Discs** – Avoid excessive forward

folds or deep backbends. Maintain a neutral spine and bend knees slightly when needed.

- **Joint Pain or Arthritis** – Modify postures to reduce pressure on wrists, knees, and hips. Use props or practice on a soft mat.
- **Pregnancy** – Consult a qualified instructor. Avoid deep forward folds, intense backbends, and lying on the stomach.
- **Menstruation** – Some prefer to avoid inversions (Downward Dog) or deep abdominal engagement during menstruation. Listen to your body and modify accordingly.

6. Keep the Neck and Spine Aligned

- Avoid straining the neck in Cobra (Bhujangasana). Keep a gentle gaze forward instead of craning the neck.
- Focus spinal length through the crown of the head and avoid collapsing into the lower back during backbends.

7. Hydration & Environment

- **Avoid dehydration** by drinking water before and after practice, but not immediately before.
- Choose a well-ventilated space with fresh air to support proper breathing.

8. Gradual Progression & Proper Technique

- Start slowly and with fewer rounds (e.g., 2-3 rounds) before increasing repetitions.
- Focus on alignment and breathing with the movements, over speed to prevent injuries.

9. End with Relaxation

- After completing Surya Namaskar, take time to rest in

Savasana (Corpse Pose) or practice deep breathing to allow the body to integrate the benefits.

By practicing with mindfulness, proper technique, and self-awareness, Surya Namaskar can be a powerful and transformative practice that enhances physical health, mental clarity, and spiritual connection.

Seated Forward Fold (Paschimottanasana)

How to Practice:

1. Sit on the floor with legs extended forward, feet flexed.
2. Inhale, lengthen the spine, reaching arms overhead.
3. Exhale, fold forward from the hips, reaching toward the feet or shins.
4. Hold for several deep breaths, allowing the torso to relax over the legs.
5. Keep the spine long and avoid rounding the back.

Benefits:

- Provides a cooling and grounding effect, counteracting the heat of summer.
- Soothes an overactive mind, calms the nervous system, and promotes deep relaxation.
- Stimulates digestion and the Small Intestine meridian, supporting the body's ability to absorb nutrients.
- Encourages introspection and surrender, balancing summer's extroverted energy.

Fish Pose (Matsyasana)

How to Practice:

1. Lie on your back with legs extended or in Lotus Pose.
2. Place hands under the hips, elbows pressing into the floor.

3. Inhale, lift the chest and arch the upper back, allowing the head to gently drop back.
4. Keep weight in the elbows and forearms rather than the crown of the head.
5. Hold for 5–10 breaths, then gently lower back down.

Benefits:

- Opens the Heart Chakra, promoting joy, emotional release, and connection.
- Stimulates the Kidney meridian, replenishing energy and preventing summer burnout.
- Expands the lungs, improving breath capacity and oxygen intake.
- Encourages circulation and energy flow, reducing stagnation.

Side Plank (Vasisthasana)

How to Practice:

1. Start in Plank Pose, shoulders stacked over wrists.
2. Shift weight to the right hand and outer edge of the right foot.
3. Stack the left foot on top, lift the left arm toward the sky, and engage the core.
4. Hold for several breaths, then switch sides.
5. For variations, lift the top leg or extend the top arm overhead.

Benefits:

- Strengthens the arms, core, and shoulders, building endurance.
- Encourages inner fire and resilience, aligning with summer's radiant energy.
- Expands the chest, fostering confidence and self-expression.

- Promotes mental focus and balance, helping to cultivate presence.

Lotus Pose (Padmasana)

How to Practice:

1. Sit with legs extended, bend one knee, and place the foot onto the opposite thigh.
2. Repeat with the other leg, placing it over the first foot.
3. Rest hands on the knees in a mudra of your choice(e.g., Chin or Gyan Mudra).
4. Maintain a tall spine and focus on slow, deep breathing.

Benefits:

- Deepens meditation and inner peace, promoting harmony with the Fire element.
- Opens the hips and encourages emotional balance.
- Grounds excessive energy while soothing the heart and nervous system.
- Supports self-reflection and spiritual awareness, fostering a sense of connection.

PRANAYAMA (BREATHING TECHNIQUES) FOR SUMMER

Breathing techniques, or pranayama, can help regulate the body's internal heat and emotional balance, especially during the intensity of summer. Two pranayama techniques are particularly useful for supporting the Heart meridian and cultivating balance:

Sheetali Pranayama (Cooling Breath)

How to Practice:

1. Sit in a comfortable position with your spine tall and shoulders relaxed.

2. Close your eyes and take a deep inhale through the nose.
3. Curl your tongue into a tube shape (if unable, purse your lips into an "O" shape instead).
4. Inhale deeply through the curled tongue or pursed lips, drawing in cool air.
5. Exhale through the same shape with cooling breath.
6. Repeat for 5–10 rounds, focusing on the cooling sensation spreading through your body.

Benefits:

- Reduces excess heat in the body, making it perfect for summer or hot climates.
- Balances the Fire element, calming the heart and soothing emotional intensity.
- Relieves stress and anxiety, promoting relaxation.
- Aids digestion and prevents heat-related ailments like acid reflux and skin irritation.

Bhramari Pranayama (Bee Breath)

How to Practice:

1. Sit in a comfortable seated posture with eyes closed and hands resting on your knees.
2. Take a deep inhale through the nose.
3. As you exhale, gently press your fingers over your ears to close them.
4. Keep your lips closed and make a soft, steady humming sound (like a bee's buzz) as you exhale.
5. Feel the vibrations resonating through your head and chest.
6. Repeat for 5–7 rounds, focusing on the calming effect on your nervous system.

Benefits:

- Soothes the nervous system, reducing stress and tension.
- Releases excess heat and cools the body.
- Clears mental clutter and enhances focus.
- Balances emotions, making it effective for summer irritability or restlessness.
- Improves sleep quality by calming the mind.

MEDITATIONS FOR SUMMER: CULTIVATING LOVE, JOY, AND INNER LIGHT

Summer is the season for joy, creativity, and emotional balance. Meditation practices focused on the Heart, and solar plexus can help us cultivate these qualities, allowing us to connect with our inner light and inspire our emotional well-being.

Heart-Centered Meditation

This meditation helps cultivate feelings of love, joy, gratitude, and compassion, aligning with the Fire element and the Heart meridian in summer. It supports emotional balance, reduces stress, and deepens your connection with yourself and others.

How to Practice:

1. Find a comfortable seated position, either on a cushion, chair, or with your back supported.
2. Close your eyes and take a few deep breaths, allowing your body to relax.
3. Place your hands over your heart center (middle of your chest) and bring your awareness to this area.
4. As you inhale, imagine a warm, golden or green light filling your heart—expanding with each breath.
5. With each exhale, allow any tension, stress, or heaviness to dissolve and release.

6. Bring to mind a person, place, or experience that fills you with gratitude and joy. Let the feeling of love expand, radiating outward from your heart.
7. Stay with this feeling for 5–10 minutes, embracing the warmth and connection.
8. When ready, gently bring your awareness back, wiggle your fingers and toes, and open your eyes slowly.

Benefits:

- Enhances emotional balance, self-love, and resilience.
- Expands compassion and connection with others.
- Reduces stress, heart tension, and supports cardiovascular health.
- Aligns with the Fire element, nurturing the Heart meridian in summer.

Solar Plexus Meditation

The Solar Plexus (Manipura Chakra) is the center of personal power, confidence, and vitality. This meditation strengthens self-trust, motivation, and enthusiasm—perfect for embracing summer's radiance and expansion.

How to Practice:

1. Sit or lie down in a comfortable, relaxed position.
2. Close your eyes and take a deep inhale through the nose, exhaling slowly through the mouth.
3. Bring your awareness to the Solar Plexus (upper abdomen, just above the navel).
4. Imagine a warm, golden sun glowing in this space, radiating heat and light.
5. As you inhale, visualize the light growing brighter, filling your entire body with strength and confidence.
6. As you exhale, imagine any doubts, fears, or insecurities dissolving into the warmth.

7. Repeat a silent affirmation, such as:*"I am strong, radiant, and confident.", "I embrace my power with joy and courage."*
8. Let this inner fire expand outward, increasing your motivation and passion for life.
9. After 5–10 minutes, bring your awareness back, open your eyes, and notice how you feel.

Benefits:

- Boosts confidence, personal power, and motivation.
- Increases vitality, enthusiasm, and clarity of purpose.
- Supports digestion and energy flow through the Small Intestine meridian.
- Helps transform self-doubt into self-trust and action.

QI GONG FOR SUMMER

"Heart Opening Lotus Flow" (Fire Element – Heart & Small Intestine)

Purpose: Summer is the season of warmth, joy, and radiance. This practice helps expand the chest, nourish the Heart meridian, and encourage emotional openness.

How to Practice:

1. Begin in a Wuji/Horse Stance – Feet wider than hip-width, knees slightly bent, spine lifting up.
2. Inhale & Open the Arms – Sweep the arms out and up, forming a circle overhead, palms facing the sky.
3. Exhale & Lower Hands to the Heart – Bring palms together at the chest, as if holding a blooming lotus flower.
4. Inhale & Expand Again – Imagine gathering joyful energy from the sun as your arms open wide.
5. Exhale & Return to the Heart – Feel warmth radiating from your chest.
6. Repeat for 8–12 breaths, letting go of stress and inviting love, laughter, and gratitude into your practice.

7. Visualize the heart glowing like the summer sun, radiating warmth and connection.

SENSORY ACTIVITIES

Sound: Embrace the Rhythms of Summer

Sunset Meditation: As the day winds down, sit quietly and meditate during a summer sunset. Listen attentively to the soothing sounds of nature—the rustling of leaves in the breeze, the gentle call of birds returning to their nests, or the distant hum of summer insects. Allow these sounds to bring you into a deep state of relaxation and mindfulness, helping you transition from the busyness of the day to a peaceful, reflective evening.

Outdoor Music: Summer is a season filled with festivals, concerts, and vibrant outdoor events. Take time to enjoy live music performances in parks or open-air venues. Whether it's a concert, a street musician, or a local festival, the joyful sounds of music in the fresh air provide a perfect way to celebrate the abundance of life during the summer months.

Sight: Soak in the Colors and Light of Summer

Outdoor Yoga: Practice yoga or exercise in a natural setting like a park, beach, or near a river. As you stretch and move, allow your eyes to take in the vast expanses of the natural world—golden sand, green trees, clear blue skies, and the expansive horizon. The beauty of the summer landscape can uplift your spirit, deepen your connection to nature, and enhance the vitality of your practice.

Nature Walks: Engage in mindful walks through parks, forests, or along rivers, and immerse yourself in the colors of summer. Take note of the vibrant hues of blooming flowers, the deep green foliage, and the colorful display of fruits and vegetables at the market. If you can, try sun gazing at sunrise or sunset to witness the breathtaking palette of colors that the sun offers during these magical times of day.

Taste: Savor the Freshness of Summer

Barbecue Party: Gather with friends and family for a summer barbecue. Grill up classic summer favorites like burgers, corn on the cob, and roasted vegetables. The rich flavors and vibrant colors of freshly prepared food offer both a feast for the eyes and the palate. As you savor each bite, be mindful of the tastes and textures that come with the season—juicy fruits, grilled vegetables, and fragrant herbs.

Seasonal Fruit Exploration: Explore the flavors of summer fruits like watermelon, strawberries, peaches, and citrus. Create refreshing fruit salads or smoothies, incorporating cooling, hydrating ingredients. If you enjoy experimenting in the kitchen, try making your own popsicles using fresh fruit juices or herbal teas for a cool, summery treat.

Smell: Engage with the Fragrance of Summer

Campfire Gathering: Spend an evening around a campfire with friends or family, enjoying the rich, smoky scent of burning wood in the air. As you relax under the starry sky, share stories, roast marshmallows, and bask in the warmth of the fire. The primal, earthy scent of a campfire is deeply grounding and connects us to the natural rhythms of the earth.

Botanical Gardens and Flower Scents: Visit a botanical garden or flower farm to experience the intoxicating aromas of blooming summer flowers like roses, lavender, and jasmine. These natural fragrances can have an uplifting effect on the mind and body, helping to ease tension and evoke positive emotions. Alternatively, create your own natural potpourri or sachets using dried flowers, citrus peels, and herbs to infuse your home with the fresh, summery scents of nature.

Touch: Connect with the Elements of Summer

Swimming in Cool Water: There's nothing more refreshing than taking a dip in a lake, river, or ocean during summer. Let the cool water envelop your body and wash away any physical or mental fatigue. Allow the sensations of water against your skin to ground you and reconnect you to your body's natural rhythms. If swimming is not an option, simply wading in cool water or walking barefoot on the beach or grass can be equally revitalizing.

Outdoor Yoga or Meditation: Practice yoga or meditation outdoors and focus on the sensations of the sun on your skin and the breeze against your body. The warmth of the sun can invigorate you, while the gentle wind can bring a sense of peace and balance. Ground yourself by feeling the earth beneath you, letting go of any tension as you breathe in the fresh, clean air.

ALIGNING WITH THE SUMMER SEASON

Summer is a season of celebration, vitality, and creativity. By engaging your senses with the natural world around you, you align yourself with the energetic flow of the season. Embrace the Fire element by connecting with others, expressing your creativity, and nourishing your body with fresh, seasonal foods. Whether it's enjoying the sunshine, engaging in joyful social gatherings, or basking in the warmth of nature, summer offers a time to ignite your inner spark, celebrate life, and feel the vibrancy of your own being.

By fully embracing the sights, sounds, tastes, smells, and sensations of summer, you can experience the true abundance and vitality that this season has to offer. Soak in the richness of life, and let the energy of summer fuel your personal growth, creativity, and joy.

A SPECIAL NOTE ON "JOMO"

The acronym for "Joy of Missing Out," JOMO, represents the pleasure derived from living in a quiet or independent way without feeling anxious about missing out on exciting or interesting events elsewhere. In today's fast-paced and hyper-connected world, where the fear of missing out (FOMO) often prevails, embracing JOMO can be a refreshing and liberating mindset, especially during the summer season.

As the days grow longer and the social calendar fills up with various activities and events, it is essential to find moments of solitude and inner peace. JOMO allows us to step back, disconnect from the constant stream of notifications, and prioritize our well-being and personal needs. It provides an opportunity to savor the simple joys of life, whether it's spending time alone in nature, engaging in creative pursuits, or relishing quiet moments of reflection and self-care.

Embracing JOMO during summer can be seen as the perfect antidote to a season that often encourages excess and constant stimulation.

By embracing the value of JOMO, we can cultivate a deeper sense of contentment, gratitude, and inner fulfillment, allowing us to fully immerse ourselves in the present moment and create a more balanced and fulfilling summer experience.

AROMATHERAPY FOR SUMMER

Aromatherapy can enhance your emotional well-being and support the energy of the Heart during summer. Certain essential oils are especially beneficial for the Heart meridian, aiding in calming, uplifting, and balancing emotions.

Here are some essential oils to consider for your summer wellness routine:

1. Rose

Rose essential oil is revered for its ability to **calm** the heart and promote **emotional balance.** Known as the "queen of oils," it helps open the heart to love and compassion, fostering a deep sense of connection and well-being.

2. Lavender

Lavender oil is widely known for its **soothing** and **calming** properties. It helps reduce **stress** and **anxiety**, making it an excellent choice for balancing emotions and supporting restful sleep, which is crucial for heart health.

3. Ylang Ylang

With its sweet, floral aroma, Ylang Ylang oil is perfect for **uplifting** the spirit and **balancing** emotions. It reduces **stress**, encourages relaxation, and fosters harmony in the heart, helping you release tension and open yourself to love and connection.

4. Bergamot

Bergamot oil has a refreshing citrus scent that can **uplift** the spirits and promote **emotional well-being.** It is highly effective in reducing **stress** and **anxiety** while promoting a **positive outlook** that supports the heart's vitality.

5. Frankincense

Frankincense oil is known for its **grounding** and **calming** effects. It can help reduce **feelings of anxiety**, promote **inner peace**, and support emotional well-being, making it beneficial for heart health.

6. Melissa (Lemon Balm)

Melissa oil has a sweet, citrusy aroma and is known for its **calming** and **uplifting** properties. It supports **emotional well-being**, reduces feelings of overwhelm, and nurtures the heart during times of stress.

USING ESSENTIAL OILS SAFELY

As with all essential oils, be sure to follow proper dilution and usage guidelines. When using citrus oils, such as Lemon and Bergamot, be cautious of photo sensitivity. Always consult a qualified aromatherapist or healthcare professional for personalized guidance, especially if you have specific health concerns. *Refer to Part 3: Chapter 8-Smell, for more on the Safe usage of essential oils

CONCLUSION

Summer invites us to connect with the radiant energy of the Fire element, embracing our inner passion, creativity, and love.

Through yoga, pranayama, meditation, Qi gong, and Aromatherapy, we can support the organs of summer-Heart and Small Intestine- and foster emotional well-being, vitality, and joy. By integrating these practices into your life, you can enhance your connection to the powerful energy of summer, allowing your heart to open fully to the beauty and possibility of the season.

May this season bring you closer to your inner light, empowering you to live with purpose, love, and enthusiasm!

P.S. You have permission to keep refining what that means to you and what brings you joy at each stage of your journey.

15
LATE SUMMER-NURTURING AND HARVEST

The Bountiful Harvest

Golden fields sway in a gentle breeze,
Earth's bounty whispers, "Nurture and ease..."
Root down deep, draw strength from the land,
Abundance is grief and gratitude, hand in hand.
Beneath the soil, steady and strong,
Earth reminds us—this is where we belong.
Nourishing bodies with balance and care,
In rhythm with nature, standing still, aware.
Through breath and movement, stillness and flow,
We weave a union that starts to grow.
Cradled in Earth's unwavering grace,
She holds our health, our wealth, our place—
A steady light for all our days.

-Erika Hawley

A TIME OF HARVEST AND HARMONY- THE EARTH ELEMENT

In Chinese Medicine, late summer represents the Earth element—a time of transition and balance. This season is about nurturing and stabilizing- a chance to embody the energy of harvest and abundance.

It is when the Earth's energy reaches its peak, offering us all an invitation to savor the fruits of the year's efforts. The Earth element is deeply connected to the Spleen (Yin organ) and Stomach (Yang organ), which govern digestion, nourishment, and the assimilation of life's experiences. It is a time to take stock of what has been created and to nurture ourselves with grounding, nourishing foods and practices.

Late summer calls for gratitude and connection with the earth's bounty. It's a time to nourish both body and spirit through self-care and earth based exercises.

By embracing this period, we can feel more connected to the present moment and balanced as we prepare for the upcoming shift into autumn.

Associations with Late Summer according to TCM:

- **Organs:** Spleen (Yin) and Stomach (Yang)
- **Sense Organ:** Mouth and lips
- **Tissues:** Muscles
- **Emotion:** Worry/Overthinking (imbalanced), Sympathy/Nurturing (balanced)
- **Color:** Yellow
- **Taste:** Sweet
- **Smell:** Fragrant
- **Energy:** Grounding, nurturing, and stability; a time of abundance and preparation for transition.

- **Seasonal Focus:** Digestion and nourishment. Supports the Spleen and Stomach's role in processing food and thoughts, turning them into Qi and blood.

EARTH ELEMENT AND THE MOUTH

The mouth and lips are associated with the Earth element, which governs the ability to nourish and sustain us physically and emotionally. During late summer, we engage the mouth and taste buds to enjoy the harvest of seasonal foods, while the lips and speech help us express gratitude and communicate our gratitude with others.

NUTRITIONAL GUIDANCE FOR LATE SUMMER: NOURISHING THE EARTH ELEMENT

Aligned with the Earth element's influence, late summer is a time for foods that are grounding, nourishing, and hydrating. These foods help balance the season's energy while supporting digestion, immunity and overall vitality as the seasons shift.

1. **Root Vegetables & Grounding Foods** *(Strengthen digestion & provide stable energy)*

- Sweet potatoes, carrots, beets, parsnips
- Pumpkin, winter squash, yams
- Turnips, rutabaga

2. **Naturally Sweet Fruits** *(Gently nourish the Spleen & reduce cravings for processed sugar)*

- Apples, pears, peaches, figs, persimmons
- Dates, apricots, grapes

3. **Whole Grains & Legumes** *(Support digestion & energy regulation)*

- Brown rice, millet, barley, quinoa

- Chickpeas, lentils, mung beans, adzuki beans

4. Lightly Cooked Vegetables *(Support the digestive fire & prevent dampness)*

- Zucchini, green beans, leeks, celery
- Cabbage, fennel, bok choy

5. Fermented & Probiotic Foods *(Enhance gut health & strengthen immunity)*

- Miso, sauerkraut, kimchi, yogurt
- Pickled vegetables, tempeh, kefir

6. Warming Herbs & Spices *(Aid digestion & promote circulation)*

- Ginger, cinnamon, turmeric, cardamom
- Fennel, nutmeg, clove

7. Mildly Warming Proteins *(Support Qi & muscle strength without burdening digestion)*

- Free-range chicken, turkey, eggs
- White fish, tofu, bone broth

8. Healthy Fats & Oils *(Support nourishment & energy balance)*

- Sesame oil, olive oil, flaxseeds
- Almonds, walnuts, sunflower seeds

9. Hydrating & Restorative Drinks *(Balance fluids & strengthen digestion)*

- Warm water with lemon, ginger tea
- Barley tea, chamomile tea

DIETARY TIPS FOR LATE SUMMER:

1. **Favor lightly cooked, easy-to-digest meals** to support the Spleen and prevent bloating.
2. **Eat small, frequent meals** rather than overloading digestion with heavy foods.
3. **Focus on naturally sweet foods** like squash, sweet potatoes, and fruits rather than processed sugar.
4. **Avoid excessive cold, raw, or greasy foods**, as they can weaken digestion and create dampness.

By aligning your diet with the Earth element, you cultivate stability, nourishment, and digestive strength as summer transitions into autumn.

BALANCING THE EARTH ELEMENT: YOGA, PRANAYAMA, MEDITATION, AND AROMATHERAPY FOR LATE SUMMER

The Earth element represents stability, grounding, and nourishment —qualities that are especially important as we transition through the late summer months. As the Earth element governs the Spleen and Stomach meridians in Chinese medicine, supporting these meridians through movement, breath, and mindfulness practices helps cultivate a sense of balance and harmony within our body and mind.

Yoga, pranayama, meditation, and aromatherapy are powerful tools to nourish and align with the Earth element, promoting physical, emotional, and energetic well-being.

Incorporating specific yoga poses can help activate and harmonize the Spleen and Stomach meridians, promoting grounding, digestion, and emotional stability.

Here are some key poses to incorporate into your practice for the Earth element:

Palm Tree Pose (Tadasana)

How to practice:

1. Stand with feet hip-width apart or together, pressing evenly into all four corners of your feet.
2. Engage the thighs and lengthen the spine, reaching the crown of your head toward the sky.
3. Relax the shoulders down and broaden the collarbones.
4. Bring your hands together at the heart and reach the arms up over head, palms facing upward, relax shoulders
5. Take slow, deep breaths, feeling the connection between your feet and the earth and the sky as you reach and lift upwards.

Benefits:

- Establishes stability and grounding, connecting you to the Earth element.
- Improves posture and body awareness.
- Enhances balance and focus, providing a strong foundation for movement.
- Supports emotional stability by encouraging presence and centeredness.

Warrior II (Virabhadrasana II)

How to practice:

1. Step your feet wide apart and turn one foot out 90 degrees.
2. Bend fwd on the other foot, making sure foot and front knee align over the ankle, keeping the back leg straight and strong.
3. Extend your arms parallel to the ground, gazing over the front fingertips.
4. Engage your core, and root down through both feet while lifting through the spine, sinking down through the hips.
5. Hold for 5-10 breaths, then switch sides.

Benefits:

- Strengthens the legs, core, and lower back.
- Encourages circulation and supports digestion by activating the Spleen and Stomach meridians.
- Enhances inner strength, stability, and resilience—ideal for seasonal transitions.
- Helps cultivate focus, determination, and emotional grounding as summer shifts into autumn.

<u>Shoulder/Bridge Pose (Kandarasana)</u>

How to practice:

1. Lie on your back with knees bent and feet hip-width apart, flat on the mat.
2. Press into your feet and upper back as you lift your hips toward the sky, engaging the glutes and thighs.
3. Clasp your hands underneath you, clasp the heels with your hands or keep your arms resting by your sides.
4. Hold the pose for 5-10 breaths, then slowly lower your hips back down.
5. Keep the neck lengthened and focus on breathing in/out at the throat center

Benefits:

- Stimulates digestion by activating the Spleen and Stomach meridians.
- Opens the chest, aiding breath and emotional balance.
- Encourages detoxification and enhances circulation.
- Provides grounding and nourishment by strengthening the back body and feet connection.

Universal Spinal Twist (Shava Udarakarshanasana)

How to practice:

1. Lie on your back and hug one knee into your chest.
2. Gently guide the bent knee across the body, allowing the opposite arm to extend outward.
3. Keep both shoulders grounded as you twist and gaze over the extended arm.
4. Hold for 5-10 breaths, then switch sides.

Benefits:

- Stimulates digestion and aids in detoxification, supporting the Spleen and Stomach meridians.
- Releases stagnation and promotes smooth energy flow, assisting in the seasonal transition.
- Opens the chest and shoulders, easing mental tension and fostering emotional balance.
- Encourages adaptability and surrender, helping shift into autumn's cooling, introspective energy.

Hare/Child's Pose (Shashankasana)

How to practice:

1. Kneel on the mat, bringing big toes together and knees apart or together.
2. Sit back onto your heels and extend your arms forward, resting your forehead on the mat or your forearms.
3. Take slow, deep breaths, softening your entire body with each exhale.
4. Stay for as long as needed, embracing the nurturing quality of the pose.

Benefits:

- Gently massages the abdominal area, aiding digestion and relaxation.
- Supports emotional grounding and releases mental tension.
- Nurtures the Earth element, promoting balance, nourishment, and calm.
- Offers a sense of safety and deep rest, helping transition into a new season with ease.

PRANAYAMA (BREATHING TECHNIQUES) FOR LATE SUMMER

Pranayama (breath work) plays a crucial role in balancing the Earth's elements. Specific breathing techniques can enhance digestion, calm the nervous system, and support the smooth flow of energy in the body. Here are two effective techniques:

Kapalabhati Pranayama (Skull Shining Breath)

How to practice:

1. Sit in a comfortable position with a tall spine, either in a cross-legged pose or on a chair with feet flat on the floor.
2. Rest your hands on your knees with palms facing upward.
3. Take a deep inhale through the nose, filling the lungs.
4. Begin rapid, forceful exhalations through the nose by contracting the lower belly (below the navel). The inhalation happens naturally between each exhale.
5. Continue this cycle for about 30 rounds, keeping a steady pace.
6. After completing one round, take a deep inhale, hold the breath for a few seconds, and then exhale slowly.
7. Repeat for 2-3 rounds, gradually increasing as you build stamina.

Benefits:

- Energizes the body and clears mental fog.

- Stimulates digestion and metabolism, supporting the Spleen and Stomach meridians.
- Removes stagnant energy and toxins through rapid exhalations.
- Improves focus and mental clarity, making it ideal for early morning practice.

Precautions:

- Avoid if pregnant, have high blood pressure, heart conditions, or respiratory issues.
- Always practice on an empty stomach.

Nadi Shodhana Pranayama (Alternate Nostril Breathing)

How to practice:

1. Sit in a comfortable meditation posture with the spine upright and shoulders relaxed.
2. Use Nasagra Mudra with your right hand (Place the index and middle fingers on the eyebrow center. Relax your hand. Use your right thumb to close your right nostril. Use your ring finger to close your left nostril)
3. Close the right nostril with the thumb and inhale slowly and deeply through the left nostril.
4. Close the left nostril with the ring finger, release the right nostril, and exhale through the right.
5. Inhale through the right nostril, then switch nostrils and exhale through the left nostril.
6. This completes one round. Continue for 5–10 rounds, maintaining slow, steady breaths.

Benefits:

- Balances the left and right hemispheres of the brain, fostering mental clarity and relaxation.

- Calms the nervous system, reducing stress and anxiety.
- Harmonizes the flow of Qi, supporting the Spleen and Stomach meridians.
- Enhances focus, emotional stability, and overall energetic balance.

Precautions:

- Avoid forceful breathing; keep the breath slow and smooth.
- If feeling dizzy, pause and return to normal breathing before continuing.

MEDITATIONS FOR GROUNDING AND EMOTIONAL BALANCE

Meditation practices are essential for cultivating a deep sense of groundedness and balance in our bodies and minds, particularly during the late summer. By focusing on the abdomen and Earth connection, we support emotional harmony and physical stability.

Grounding Meditation

How to practice:

1. Find a quiet space where you can sit comfortably, either on the floor or in a chair with your feet firmly planted.
2. Close your eyes and take a few deep breaths, inhaling through the nose and exhaling through the mouth.
3. Visualize roots extending from the base of your spine (or from your feet, if seated in a chair), reaching deep into the Earth.
4. Imagine drawing nourishing energy from the Earth up through these roots, filling your body with a sense of stability, calm, and support.
5. With each exhale, release any tension, stress, or scattered thoughts down through the roots, allowing them to be absorbed and transformed by the Earth.

6. Continue breathing deeply for 5-10 minutes, feeling grounded, steady, and present in your body.
7. When ready, gently open your eyes and take a moment to notice the sense of calm and connection before resuming your day.

Benefits:

- Promotes stability and inner strength.
- Reduces anxiety and overthinking, especially helpful in times of transition or stress.
- Enhances focus, presence, and embodiment.

Centering Meditation

How to practice:

1. Sit in a comfortable position with your spine upright, hands resting on your lower abdomen.
2. Take a few slow, deep breaths, directing your awareness to the center of your body—the area just below the navel.
3. Imagine a warm, golden light forming at this center, gently expanding with each inhale and settling with each exhale.
4. Feel this nurturing energy radiating outward, bringing balance and harmony to your entire being.
5. If your mind wanders, gently return your focus to the warmth in your abdomen, trusting in the body's natural wisdom.
6. Continue this practice for 5-10 minutes, feeling aligned, centered, and at ease.
7. When you're ready, take a few deeper breaths, then slowly open your eyes, carrying this sense of stability and balance with you.

Benefits:

- Supports digestion and emotional stability, aligning with the Spleen and Stomach meridians.
- Calms an overactive mind, reducing worry and stress.
- Enhances self-awareness and resilience.

QI GONG FOR SUPPORTING THE EARTH ELEMENT

"Earth Centering Qi Flow" (Earth Element – Spleen & Stomach)

Purpose: This practice enhances digestion, stability, and inner balance.

How to Practice:

1. Stand with Feet Hip-Width Apart – Knees soft, hands resting on the lower abdomen (Dantian).
2. Inhale & Scoop Energy Up – Slowly raise your arms, palms facing up, as if lifting a golden ball of energy from the earth to your heart.
3. Exhale & Press Energy Down – Turn the palms downward and gently push energy back to the earth, grounding yourself.
4. Repeat for 5–10 rounds, moving at a steady, peaceful pace.
5. Imagine the earth beneath you providing stability and nourishment, filling you with strength and centeredness.

SENSORY ACTIVITIES

Sight: Witness the Subtle Changes in Nature

Leisurely Walks in Nature: Take time for slow, mindful walks in your neighborhood or a local park. Late summer foliage often transitions from vibrant greens to warmer shades of yellow, orange, and even red. This subtle shift in color is nature's invitation to reflect on change, growth, and the passage of time. Watch how the landscape evolves as you observe the transition from summer's fullness to the quiet anticipation of autumn.

Sunlit Reflections on Water: Spend time near a lake, river, or pond to witness the soft play of sunlight on the surface of the water. The shifting reflections of trees, clouds, and sky create a serene and calming environment. Allow your eyes to follow the gentle ripples in the water, taking in the peaceful, natural beauty.

Sound: Connecting with Nature's Melody

Late Summer Sounds: Late summer is marked by the distinct sounds of nature winding down. Insects, like crickets and cicadas, hum in the background as birds begin to change their migration patterns. The rustling of leaves and the occasional breeze add a melodic touch to the day. Spend time in a park or forest and listen to the sounds of late summer. Allow the natural symphony to bring you into a calm, meditative state.

Sunset Sounds: As the day shifts into the evening, find a peaceful spot to listen to the rhythmic chirping of crickets or the gentle rustling of leaves in the wind. The sounds of late summer nights are deeply soothing, offering a moment of relaxation and stillness as the world prepares to cool down.

Taste: Savoring the Harvest of Late Summer

Seasonal Fruits and Vegetables: Late summer is a time to indulge in the abundance of fresh, seasonal produce. Savor the flavors of juicy peaches, ripe tomatoes, corn on the cob, and sweet melons. These fruits and vegetables not only nourish the body but provide a perfect balance of sweetness that aligns with the energy of the Earth element, which is associated with late summer. Incorporate them into salads, salsas, or grilled dishes to celebrate the flavors of the season.

Refreshing Summer Desserts: Experiment with making fruit-based desserts like fruit salad, sorbet, or popsicles. These treats are both cooling and hydrating, offering a burst of sweetness to awaken the senses while supporting your body's need for light, refreshing foods.

Smell: Immersing Yourself in the Earth's Fragrance

The Fragrance of Late Summer: Take deep, slow breaths of the warm, earthy scents that define late summer. The aroma of ripening fruit, sun-warmed soil, and flowering herbs fills the air. If possible, visit a local orchard or farmer's market to experience the fresh, fragrant air of harvest time. These smells help ground the spirit and connect you to the earth's abundance.

Create Aromatic Blends: Surround yourself with the scents of summer by creating natural potpourri or sachets using dried flowers like lavender, rosemary, and chamomile, along with citrus peels or spices like cinnamon and cloves. These seasonal fragrances will infuse your home with the sweet, soothing aromas of late summer, enhancing a sense of calm and contentment.

Touch: Grounding Yourself in the Warmth of Late Summer

Outdoor Activities: Engage in activities that allow you to feel the warmth of late summer sunshine on your skin. Whether it's a picnic in the park, yoga in the garden, or spending time gardening, take the opportunity to bask in the light and soak up the gentle warmth of the sun. Feel the earth beneath your feet, the coolness of the grass against your skin, or the softness of the sand during a beach walk. These tactile experiences can help you stay grounded as the season transitions.

Enjoy Late Summer Evenings: As the weather starts to cool, late summer evenings offer the perfect opportunity to enjoy the fresh air. Spend time outdoors, feeling the gentle evening breeze on your face and the soft grass or sand beneath your feet. Allow the sensations of touch—whether it's the texture of your surroundings or the warmth of the air—to bring you into a state of peaceful relaxation.

AROMATHERAPY FOR THE EARTH ELEMENT: ESSENTIAL OILS FOR GROUNDING AND DIGESTIVE HEALTH

1. Ginger

Ginger essential oil is warming and promotes healthy digestion. It stimulates the **Spleen** and **Stomach meridians**, enhancing the flow of **Qi** and helping to soothe digestive discomfort.

2. Peppermint

Peppermint essential oil has a refreshing, cooling effect that supports digestion and calms the **Spleen** and **Stomach meridians**, making it perfect for digestive support.

3. Fennel

Fennel essential oil promotes healthy digestion and harmonizes the **Spleen** and **Stomach meridians.** It has a sweet, anise-like aroma that supports detoxification and emotional balance.

4. Lemon

Lemon essential oil is cleansing and uplifting, invigorating the **Spleen** and **Stomach meridians.** It promotes **mental clarity** and supports digestion.

5. Cardamom

Cardamom essential oil has digestive benefits, promoting the health of the **Spleen** and **Stomach meridians.** Its warm, spicy aroma is uplifting and stimulating.

6. Sweet Orange

Sweet orange essential oil supports the **Spleen** and **Stomach meridians**, helping to harmonize digestion and boost **energy**.

7. Cinnamon

Cinnamon essential oil possesses **warming** and **stimulating** properties that invigorate the **Spleen** and **Stomach meridians**, promoting healthy digestion and enhancing Qi circulation.

USING ESSENTIAL OILS SAFELY

As with all essential oils, be sure to follow proper dilution and usage guidelines. When using citrus oils, such as Lemon and Bergamot, be cautious of photo sensitivity. Always consult a qualified aromatherapist or healthcare professional for personalized guidance, especially if you have specific health concerns. *Refer to Part 3: Chapter 8-Smell, for more on the Safe usage of essential oils

CONCLUSION: HARMONY AND BALANCE IN LATE SUMMER

Late summer is a time to celebrate abundance, connect with the earth, and find balance as we move from the outward, expansive energy of summer toward the more introspective energy of autumn.

By engaging all of your senses in practices that connect you with the season—whether through savoring the harvest, enjoying the sights and sounds of nature, or grounding yourself through touch—you can cultivate a sense of inner peace and stability.

Embrace the Earth element by nourishing your body with sweet, grounding foods, staying hydrated, and practicing self-care. Late summer invites you to enjoy the present moment, express gratitude, and find harmony in the abundance around you. By doing so, you align with the rhythms of nature, allowing yourself to feel stable, nourished, and ready to embrace the change of seasons ahead.

16 AUTUMN-RELEASE AND TRANSFORMATION

The Dance of Letting Go

Leaves cascade in an autumnal shower,
Crisp air whispers, surrender...
to nature's power.
In release, transformation takes flight,
Embracing the change,
finding solace in the night.
The trees reveal a hidden scene,
How beautiful it is to be fully seen!
Like precious metal, refined and pure,
The essence of each element endures.
Breathe deep, let your soul expand with the air,
Activate the lungs, invite cleansing with care.
In movement, there is strength at the core,
A radiant jewel—timeless, evermore.

—**Erika Hawley**

AUTUMN: A SEASON OF LETTING GO AND REFLECTION

In Chinese Medicine, autumn represents the Metal element, a time for release, refinement, and clarity. This is the season when nature encourages us to let go of what no longer serves us, just as trees shed their leaves in preparation for the stillness of winter.

Autumn is a time for harvest, both in the literal sense of gathering crops and in the metaphorical sense of reflecting on the fruits of our labor and life's experiences.

The Metal element governs the Lungs (Yin organ) and the Large Intestine (Yang organ). These organs are linked to the processes of elimination—breathing in fresh air and expelling waste, or taking in the good Qi and letting go of the bad Qi.

In autumn, we are invited to clear out what no longer serves us, allowing space for renewal and introspection. This is a time to nourish the body with foods that support the lungs and digestive system, to release emotional baggage, and to reflect on our journey thus far.

Associations with Autumn according to TCM:

- **Organs:** Lungs (Yin) and Large Intestine (Yang)
- **Sense Organ:** Nose
- **Tissues:** Skin
- **Emotion:** Grief/Sadness (imbalanced), Acceptance/Letting Go (balanced)
- **Color:** White
- **Taste:** Pungent
- **Smell:** Rotten
- **Energy:** Reflection, letting go, and inspiration; a time of harvest and release.
- **Seasonal Focus:** Respiratory and elimination health. Supports the Lungs' role in breath and the Large

Intestine's role in letting go of waste, both physical and emotional.

METAL ELEMENT AND THE NOSE

The nose is the sensory organ linked to Autumn and the Metal element, playing a vital role in respiration, purification, and our connection to the world around us through scent.

Breathing deeply in crisp autumn air can be a powerful way to support the Lungs, while aromatherapy, mindful breath work, and spending time in nature can enhance our ability to take in life fully.

Scents like eucalyptus, frankincense, and pine help open the nasal passages, supporting clear breathing and emotional clarity. As we embrace the cool, contracting energy of autumn, we are reminded that just as each breath nourishes us, the ability to exhale and release is equally essential for creating space for new inspiration, balance, and resilience.

NUTRITIONAL RECOMMENDATIONS FOR AUTUMN: NOURISHING THE METAL ELEMENT

In keeping with the energy of the Metal element, autumn calls for foods that nourish, ground, and hydrate. These quality foods support the lungs and digestive system, helping to balance the body and offer valuable nutrition to support us as we transition into cooler weather. Focus on warming, hydrating, and easily digestible foods to help maintain harmony.

This is a season of dryness and transition, making it essential to eat moistening, warming, and immune-supporting foods to protect the respiratory system, strengthen digestion, and prepare for the colder months ahead.

1. Moistening & Lung-Nourishing Fruits

(Combat dryness, support respiratory health)

- Pears, apples, persimmons
- Grapes, figs, pomegranates
- Bananas, white peaches, apricots

2. Root Vegetables & Hearty Squashes

(Grounding, warming, and immune-boosting)

- Sweet potatoes, carrots, beets, parsnips
- Pumpkins, winter squash, butternut squash
- Turnips, rutabaga, daikon radish

3. Whole Grains & Fiber-Rich Foods

(Support digestion & regulate elimination)

- Brown rice, oats, millet, barley
- Quinoa, buckwheat, amaranth
- Lentils, chickpeas, black beans

4. Fermented & Gut-Healing Foods

(Support immunity & digestive health)

- Sauerkraut, kimchi, miso, pickled vegetables
- Yogurt, kefir, tempeh, natto

5. Immune-Boosting Herbs & Spices

(Warm the body, clear phlegm, and protect the lungs)

- Ginger, cinnamon, cloves, nutmeg
- Garlic, onions, leeks, scallions
- Turmeric, fennel, star anise

6. Lightly Cooked Greens & Cruciferous Vegetables

(Clear toxins, strengthen the immune system)

- Cabbage, Brussels sprouts, cauliflower
- Kale, bok choy, Swiss chard
- Mustard greens, watercress

7. Healthy Fats & Oils

(Moisturize the lungs and skin, provide energy balance)

- Avocados, sesame oil, olive oil
- Almonds, walnuts, pine nuts, flaxseeds

8. Warming Proteins

(Support Qi and prepare for colder months)

- Free-range chicken, turkey, duck
- Wild-caught fish, eggs
- Bone broth, tofu

9. Hydrating & Restorative Teas

(Support lung health, prevent dryness, and warm the body)

- Ginger tea, cinnamon tea, chai
- Licorice root tea, honey-lemon tea
- Barley tea, white tea

AUTUMN EATING TIPS:

1. **Eat warm, lightly cooked meals** to protect digestion and keep the body warm.
2. **Incorporate lung-moistening foods** like pears, nuts, and healthy oils to prevent dryness.
3. **Reduce raw, cold, and overly spicy foods,** as they can weaken digestion and create internal dryness.
4. **Enjoy warming soups and broths** to build immunity and strengthen the body for winter.

By following TCM's seasonal eating wisdom, you can strengthen your lungs, support digestion, and build resilience during the cooler, drier months of autumn.

REFINING THE METAL ELEMENT: YOGA, PRANAYAMA, MEDITATION, AND AROMATHERAPY FOR AUTUMN

As we transition into autumn, the Metal element comes into focus, associated with the Lungs and Large Intestine meridians in Chinese medicine. Autumn is a season of letting go, reflection, and renewal, and it is important to support the Lungs for emotional and physical clarity. Yoga, pranayama, meditation, and aromatherapy are invaluable tools for harmonizing the body's energy, enhancing respiratory health, supporting digestion, and fostering inner peace.

Here are some key poses to incorporate into your practice:

Boat Pose (Naukasana)

How to practice:

1. Sit on the floor with your legs extended in front of you.
2. Bend your knees and lift your feet off the floor, bringing your shins parallel to the ground.
3. Extend your arms forward, parallel to the floor, with palms facing each other.
4. If possible, straighten your legs into a "V" shape, keeping your core engaged and chest lifted.
5. Hold for 5–10 breaths, then slowly lower your feet back down with control.

Benefits:

- Strengthens the core and stimulates digestive organs, supporting the Large Intestine meridian.
- Improves stability and balance, aligning with autumn's grounding energy.

- Helps detoxify by activating digestion and promoting the release of what no longer serves.

Triangle Pose (Trikonasana)

How to practice:

1. Stand with your feet 3–4 feet apart, right foot turned out 90 degrees and left foot slightly inward.
2. Extend your arms parallel to the floor, palms facing down.
3. Reach your right hand forward and lower it to your shin, ankle, or the floor outside your right foot.
4. Extend your left arm straight up, keeping your gaze at your top hand or forward.
5. Hold for 5–8 breaths, then switch sides.

Benefits:

- Expands the chest and opens the Lung meridian, improving breathing capacity.
- Stretches the side body and enhances circulation, assisting in seasonal detoxification.
- Encourages mental clarity and balance, aligning with autumn's reflective nature.

Supported Shoulder/Bridge Pose (Kandarasana)

How to practice:

1. Lie on your back with knees bent and feet hip-width apart, flat on the floor.
2. Place a yoga block or bolster under your sacrum for support.
3. Press your feet into the ground, lengthen the back of your neck and slowly begin lifting your hips slightly as you relax your upper back into the floor.
4. Open your hips and torso- breathe deeply in and out with a focus on the throat area, keeping your arms by your sides.

5. Hold for 8–10 breaths before slowly lowering down- head to tail.

Benefits:

- Opens the chest, improving lung capacity and circulation.
- Stimulates digestion and supports the Large Intestine meridian, assisting in detoxification.
- Encourages emotional release and relaxation, countering autumn's tendency for grief or introspection.

<u>Seated Half Spinal Twist (Ardha Matsyendrasana)</u>

How to practice:

1. Sit with legs extended, then bend your right knee and cross it over your left leg, placing the foot flat on the floor.
2. Bend your left knee or keep the left leg extended.
3. Place your right hand behind you for support and bring your left elbow to the outside of your right knee.
4. Inhale to lengthen the spine, exhale to twist deeper, looking over your right shoulder.
5. Hold for 5–8 breaths, then switch sides.

Benefits:

- Stimulates digestion and elimination, activating the Large Intestine meridian.
- Helps detoxify the body and support the natural process of seasonal transition.
- Encourages emotional release, promoting the ability to "let go" of stagnant energy and old patterns.

<u>Relaxation Pose (Savasana)</u>

How to practice:

1. Lie flat on your back with arms at your sides, palms facing up.
2. Allow your legs to relax, feet falling naturally outward.
3. Close your eyes and focus on deep, steady breathing.
4. Stay in the pose for 5–10 minutes, allowing full integration of your practice.

Benefits:

- Supports the Metal element by allowing energy to flow freely and settle into balance.
- Encourages introspection and emotional equilibrium, essential during this season of change.
- Promotes deep rest and nervous system regulation, essential for seasonal adaptation.

PRANAYAMA (BREATHING TECHNIQUES) FOR AUTUMN: CLEARING THE LUNGS AND BALANCING THE BODY

Inhale: Hold: Let Go – 4:7:8 Breathing

Purpose: This technique helps nourish the lungs, ease feelings of sadness or grief, and promote relaxation and emotional release. The extended exhalation supports the natural "letting go" process that aligns with autumn's energy of transformation.

How to Practice:

1. Find a comfortable seated or reclined position. Keep your spine straight and shoulders relaxed.
2. Close your eyes and take a deep inhale through your nose, filling your lungs completely.
3. Inhale deeply for 4 counts, feeling your chest expand.
4. Hold the breath for 7 counts, allowing oxygen to circulate and settle within your body.
5. Exhale slowly for 8 counts, releasing tension and stagnant energy.

6. Repeat for 5–10 rounds, gradually deepening your breath.

Benefits:

- Strengthens lung capacity and improves oxygen circulation.
- Activates the parasympathetic nervous system, reducing stress and promoting relaxation.
- Supports emotional release, helping process grief and embrace seasonal changes.

Nadi Shodhana Pranayama (Alternate Nostril Breathing)

Purpose: This traditional yogic breath work balances the nervous system, harmonizes both hemispheres of the brain, and enhances mental clarity. It is particularly effective for clearing stagnant Qi in the Lung meridian and balancing all 12 main meridians of the body.

How to Practice:

1. Sit comfortably with your spine straight and shoulders relaxed.
2. Use Nasagra Mudra with your right hand (Place the index and middle fingers on the eyebrow center. Relax your hand-Use your right thumb to close your right nostril-Use your ring finger to close your left nostril)
3. Close the right nostril with your thumb and inhale deeply through the left nostril.
4. Close the left nostril with your ring finger, release the right nostril, and exhale through the right.
5. Inhale through the right nostril, then close it, releasing the left nostril to exhale.
6. Continue alternating nostrils for 5–10 rounds, ensuring each breath remains slow and controlled.

Benefits:

- Clears the lungs and sinuses, enhancing respiratory health.

- Balances both the sympathetic (active) and parasympathetic (calm) nervous systems.
- Harmonizes the flow of Qi throughout the meridians, encouraging emotional stability.
- Promotes clarity, focus, and a sense of grounding during seasonal shifts.

MEDITATIONS FOR AUTUMN: GROUNDING AND CULTIVATING CLARITY

Autumn invites us to slow down and reflect, making it an ideal time for meditation practices that help cultivate groundedness, stability, and clarity. By focusing on the Lungs and the Metal element, we can strengthen our emotional resilience and embrace the beauty of the season's transitions.

Grounding Meditation

Purpose:

This meditation helps anchor the body and mind, fostering stability and emotional balance as we navigate the shifts of autumn. The visualization strengthens our connection to the Earth, reinforcing our foundation and resilience.

How to practice:

1. Find a quiet space where you can sit comfortably, either on the floor or in a chair with your feet firmly planted.
2. Close your eyes and take a few deep breaths, inhaling through the nose and exhaling through the mouth.
3. Visualize roots extending from the base of your spine (or from your feet, if seated in a chair), reaching deep into the Earth.
4. Imagine drawing nourishing energy from the Earth up through these roots, filling your body with a sense of stability, calm, and support.

5. With each exhale, release any tension, stress, or scattered thoughts down through the roots, allowing them to be absorbed and transformed by the Earth.
6. Continue breathing deeply for 5-10 minutes, feeling grounded, steady, and present in your body.
7. When ready, gently open your eyes and take a moment to notice the sense of calm and connection before resuming your day.

Benefits:

- Promotes stability and inner strength.
- Reduces anxiety and overthinking, especially helpful in times of transition or stress.
- Enhances focus, presence, and embodiment.

Mantra Meditation

Purpose:

Chanting mantras, especially "Om" (AUM), helps clear the mind, balance the body's energy, and enhance respiratory health. The vibration stimulates the head, chest, and lungs, promoting clarity and a sense of peace, which is especially valuable as the air becomes crisp and the energy of the season turns inward.

How to Practice:

1. Sit comfortably in a quiet place with your spine tall and shoulders relaxed.
2. Take a few deep breaths, inhaling through the nose and exhaling through the mouth.
3. Begin chanting the mantra "Om" (AUM) slowly and intentionally.
4. As you chant, feel the vibrations moving through different areas of the body: "A" resonates in the belly and chest. "U"

vibrates through the throat and upper chest. "M" hums within the center of the head and crown behind the eyes.

5. Extend any of the syllables—especially "M"—to deepen resonance and presence.
6. Repeat for 5–10 minutes, focusing on the sound and the feeling in your body.
7. If preferred, place one hand on your chest to feel the vibrations and enhance lung awareness.
8. When finished, sit in silence for a few moments, absorbing the energy of the practice before slowly opening your eyes.

Benefits:

- Supports lung health by opening the respiratory passages.
- Promotes clarity, emotional strength, and inner peace.
- Aligns with the Metal element by refining breath and energy flow.
- Encourages mindfulness and presence, helping to embrace the transitions of the season.

QI GONG FOR AUTUMN: SUPPORTING LUNG HEALTH AND EMOTIONAL CLARITY

"Lung Cleansing Breath" (Metal Element – Lungs & Large Intestine)

Purpose: This practice strengthens the Lungs, enhances breath control, and helps process grief or emotional stagnation.

How to Practice:

1. Stand with Hands on the Lower Belly – Feet shoulder-width apart, breathing deeply.
2. Inhale & Open the Arms – Raise the arms to the sides at shoulder height, opening the chest and taking in fresh energy.
3. Exhale & Cross the Arms – Sweep the arms in front of the chest, as if "hugging" yourself while exhaling fully.

4. Inhale & Open Again – Expand the arms outward, filling the lungs completely.
5. Repeat for 6–10 breaths, emphasizing deep, slow exhales to release old energy.
6. Envision breathing in crisp autumn air and exhaling any heaviness, just as leaves fall effortlessly from a tree.

SENSORY ACTIVITIES

Sight: Immerse Yourself in the Colors of Autumn

Leaf Peeping Hike: I just love that name, "Leaf Peeping" lol... it is popularly used in the eastern US, a term used when going on a walk or drive to see the changing leaves. For this exercise: Take a leisurely hike (or drive) in the woods to witness the stunning transformation of foliage. The trees, once lush and green, now don vibrant shades of red, orange, and gold. This shift symbolizes the transition from the abundance of summer to the introspection of autumn. Pause to admire the patterns of fallen leaves and reflect on the beauty of change and what that means to you at this time in life.

Outdoor Photography: Bring your camera or phone to capture the breathtaking colors of autumn. Focus on the textures of fallen leaves, bare branches, and the contrasting colors in the landscape. Through this lens, you can create lasting memories that celebrate the impermanence and transformation of the season.

Sound: Listen to the Whispers of Autumn

Crunchy Leaf Walk: Take a mindful walk through the park or along wooded trails, this time, paying close attention to the sounds beneath your feet. The satisfying crunch of dry leaves as you walk is one of autumn's unique sensory pleasures. Let the sound of rustling leaves help you stay grounded and present in the moment, fully embracing the season of letting go.

Autumn's Natural Symphony: The fall season is filled with the subtle sounds of nature preparing for winter—gentle winds, distant calls of migratory birds, and the rustle of branches swaying in the breeze. Spend some time outdoors, particularly during early mornings or late afternoons, when the air is crisp and still. Allow the peaceful sounds of autumn to deepen your sense of calm and reflection.

Taste: Savor the Flavors of the Harvest

Apple Orchard Visit: Autumn is the season of harvest, and one of the best ways to immerse yourself in this energy is by visiting a local apple orchard. Take time to pick apples directly from the trees and taste the freshness of the fruit. Savor the sweetness of apples, apple cider, and seasonal treats like apple pies and tarts. These flavors represent the essence of autumn, nourishing both the body and spirit.

Autumn-Inspired Cooking: Experiment with hearty soups, roasted vegetables, and baked goods infused with warming spices like cinnamon, nutmeg, and cloves. Pumpkin, squash, and root vegetables are staples of the season, offering comfort and nourishment. Prepare a seasonal meal that celebrates the flavors of autumn and connects you with the energy of harvest.

Smell: Breathe in the Earth's Aroma

Pumpkin Patch Exploration: Take a trip to a pumpkin patch, where the earthy, damp scent of soil and the sweet, fragrant pumpkins fill the air. Wander among the fields, breathing in the natural aromas of the harvest. The smell of the earth itself evokes the essence of autumn—nourishing, grounding, and full of potential.

Seasonal Aromas at Home: Bring the scent of autumn into your home by simmering a homemade potpourri of cinnamon sticks, cloves, orange peels, and star anise on the stove. Alternatively, light a candle or use essential oils like cedar wood, clove, or cinnamon to create a warm and inviting atmosphere that celebrates the harvest season.

Touch: Ground Yourself in the Sensations of Autumn

Cozy Blanket Snuggle: As the temperature drops, embrace the warmth and comfort of autumn by wrapping yourself in a soft, cozy blanket. Snuggle up on the couch, enjoy the cooler breeze coming through the window, and feel the comforting texture of the fabric against your skin. This simple act of self-care helps you embrace the changing seasons and offers a sense of warmth and security.

Outdoor Activities: Autumn's cool temperatures make it the perfect time to enjoy outdoor activities that engage your sense of touch. Whether it's raking leaves, gathering acorns, or simply walking barefoot on the grass, take time to connect with the tactile sensations of nature. Feel the crisp air on your skin, the texture of fallen leaves beneath your feet, and the soft earth in your hands as you prepare for the stillness of winter.

AROMATHERAPY FOR AUTUMN: ESSENTIAL OILS TO SUPPORT THE METAL ELEMENT

Essential oils can support the Lungs, immune health, and emotional well-being during the autumn season. Aromatherapy can help balance the Metal element and clear emotional and physical blockages, helping you stay grounded, focused, and resilient.

Here are some essential oils to incorporate into your autumn sensory-care routine:

1. Cinnamon

Cinnamon has a **warming** and **comforting** aroma that helps boost **immunity**, promote **circulation**, and stimulate digestion.

2. Clove

Clove is **antimicrobial** and supports **respiratory health.** It also helps alleviate cold and flu symptoms, making it ideal for boosting immunity during autumn's shift in temperatures.

3. Ginger

Ginger's warming and invigorating properties help **stimulate digestion** and relieve nausea, supporting both the **Spleen** and **Stomach meridians.** Its uplifting aroma can also help improve mood and energy.

4. Eucalyptus

Eucalyptus has powerful **respiratory support** properties, helping clear congestion and improve breathing. It is ideal for supporting the **Lungs** and promoting clearer airways during the cooler months.

5. Frankincense

Frankincense is deeply **grounding** and **calming**, helping to reduce **stress** and anxiety. It supports emotional well-being and can help clear emotional blockages, promoting a sense of peace and emotional clarity.

6. Sweet Orange

Sweet orange oil has a **bright, uplifting** aroma that enhances mood and promotes a sense of warmth and comfort. It supports **digestion** and brings emotional balance during the autumn season.

7. Nutmeg

Nutmeg's soothing and **relaxing** properties help relieve muscle tension and promote calm, aiding in the release of physical and emotional tension during the change of season.

8. Vetiver

Vetiver is a deeply **grounding** oil that helps reduce feelings of **anxiety** and **overwhelm.** Its calming aroma creates a sense of emotional stability, making it ideal for the autumn transition.

9. Cedarwood

Cedar wood has a **comforting** and **grounding** aroma that promotes relaxation and supports **respiratory health.** It's especially helpful for calming the mind and easing into restful sleep.

10. Rosemary

Rosemary is invigorating and **stimulating**, enhancing **mental clarity** and **focus**. It also supports **circulation** and **digestion**, making it an ideal choice for autumn wellness.

USING ESSENTIAL OILS SAFELY

As with all essential oils, be sure to follow proper dilution and usage guidelines. When using citrus oils, such as Lemon and Bergamot, be cautious of photo sensitivity. Always consult a qualified aromatherapist or healthcare professional for personalized guidance, especially if you have specific health concerns. *Refer to Part 3: Chapter 8- Smell, for more on the Safe usage of essential oils

CONCLUSION: EMBRACE AUTUMN'S GIFTS OF CHANGE AND REFLECTION

Autumn is a season of letting go, reflection, and nourishment. It invites us to release what no longer serves us and make space for what is to come. By engaging our senses and aligning with the Metal element, we can honor this time of transition, finding clarity, balance, and emotional renewal. Through mindful activities like savoring seasonal flavors, enjoying nature's sights and sounds, and nourishing our bodies with grounding foods, we can fully immerse ourselves in the richness of autumn and prepare for the stillness of winter.

Embrace autumn's energy by reflecting on the abundance in your life, releasing emotional baggage, and finding peace in the beauty of impermanence. Through this practice, you can tap into the wisdom of the season, fostering a deep connection with the cycles of nature and preparing for the quiet introspection that lies ahead.

17
WINTER-STILLNESS AND REFLECTION

The Serenity of Silence

Snowflakes descend softly in tranquil grace,
Water's presence stills in an icy embrace.
Reaching to find center within,
Winter's hush whispers as the light grows dim.
Beneath frozen earth, deep rivers remain,
Silent yet flowing, in wisdom's domain.
In harmony with stillness, the quiet light of the day,
We find renewal in small and deliberate ways.
Diving into the depths of Being,
Where wisdom stirs, my soul receiving.
Held by the hush, embraced by the night,
We awaken to truth in winter's soft light.
A season of listening, of rest, and release,
Where silence itself becomes a source of peace.

-Erika Hawley

Winter: A time of Embracing Stillness and Renewal

In Chinese Medicine, winter is closely associated with the Water element, a time of introspection, restoration, and deep replenishment.

This season is considered a time to conserve energy, reflect on the past year, and rest in preparation for the more active energy of spring. The Kidneys (Yin organ) and the Bladder (Yang organ) govern the Water element, and they are responsible for storing the body's vital energy (Qi) and supporting the nervous system.

Winter encourages us to slow down and turn inward. It is a time for self-care, nourishment, and reflection, allowing us to recharge our internal reserves and build the strength needed for the year ahead. Just as nature retreats during this time, we too can embrace the natural rhythms of winter, slowing down to honor the stillness and find comfort in the quietude.

In winter, the peaceful atmosphere offers the perfect opportunity for deep listening, whether it's the quiet sounds of a snowfall or the soft rustling of wind through trees. Allow the stillness of the season to deepen your connection to your inner wisdom.

Associations with Winter according to TCM:

- **Organs:** Kidneys (Yin) and Bladder (Yang)
- **Sense Organ:** Ears
- **Tissues:** Bones
- **Emotion:** Fear (imbalanced), Wisdom/Willpower (balanced)
- **Color:** Blue/Black
- **Taste:** Salty
- **Smell:** Putrid
- **Energy:** Rest, introspection, and conservation; a time to store energy and replenish resources.
- **Seasonal Focus:** Deep nourishment and restoration.

Supports the Kidneys' role in storing Jing (essence) which governs vitality, longevity, and resilience.

WATER ELEMENT AND THE EARS

The Water element governs the ears (sense organ) and is associated with qualities like stillness, reflection, and wisdom. The ears are symbolic of our ability to listen—both to the world around us and to our inner selves.

Winter teaches us that true strength lies in quietude and receptivity. Just as a still body of water reflects the sky, deep listening allows us to perceive subtle insights, reflections, unspoken truths, and the wisdom attained from witnessing in silence.

Sound healing practices, such as chanting, listening to flowing water, singing bowls, or deep vibrational tones, can harmonize the Water element as well, soothing the nervous system and restoring balance. Gentle listening-based meditations or spending time in nature absorbing the quietude of winter help refine our ability to hear not just words, but the deeper resonance of life itself.

By honoring the Water element and our sense of hearing, we cultivate inner wisdom, resilience, and the ability to move fluidly with change.

NUTRITIONAL RECOMMENDATIONS FOR WINTER: NOURISHING THE WATER ELEMENT

Winter's cold temperatures demand warming, nourishing, and hydrating foods that help the body conserve energy and maintain internal warmth. Foods during this time should be grounded, easy to digest, and rich in nutrients. Slow-cooked meals, root vegetables, and warming spices are ideal for supporting digestion, boosting immunity, and providing comfort during the colder months.

This season calls for warming, nourishing, and deeply restorative foods to support the body's core energy, strengthen immunity, and protect against the cold.

1. Warming & Hearty Root Vegetables

(Provide grounding energy and support digestion)

- Sweet potatoes, yams, parsnips
- Beets, carrots, turnips
- Rutabaga, daikon radish

2. Slow-Cooked Whole Grains

(Strengthen digestion and provide sustained energy)

- Brown rice, wild rice, black rice
- Oats, millet, quinoa, barley
- Amaranth, buckwheat

3. Legumes & Fiber-Rich Foods

(Support kidney function and nourish blood)

- Black beans, kidney beans, lentils
- Chickpeas, adzuki beans, navy beans
- Mung beans, split peas

4. Dark Leafy Greens & Cruciferous Vegetables

(Rich in minerals and antioxidants for winter vitality)

- Kale, collard greens, mustard greens
- Brussels sprouts, broccoli, cabbage
- Bok choy, Swiss chard

5. High-Quality Animal Proteins & Bone Broths

(Deeply nourish the kidneys and support immune strength)

- Grass-fed beef, lamb, bison, duck
- Free-range chicken, turkey, eggs
- Wild-caught salmon, sardines, anchovies
- Bone broth, organ meats (kidney, liver)

6. Sea Vegetables & Mineral-Rich Foods

(Strengthen kidney function and provide essential nutrients)

- Nori, wakame, kombu, dulse
- Seaweed-based broths and soups
- Miso, tofu, tempeh

7. Healthy Fats & Warming Oils

(Provide internal warmth and lubricate joints in cold weather)

- Avocados, sesame oil, coconut oil
- Nuts (walnuts, almonds, chestnuts)
- Seeds (chia, flax, pumpkin, sesame)

8. Kidney-Tonic Fruits

(Support hydration and gentle detoxification)

- Blackberries, blueberries, cherries
- Pomegranates, figs, dates
- Persimmons, pears, citrus fruits

9. Warming Spices & Herbal Tonics

(Boost circulation, digestion, and immunity)

- Ginger, cinnamon, cloves, nutmeg
- Garlic, onions, leeks, scallions
- Star anise, black pepper, turmeric

10. Nourishing Teas & Hydrating Drinks

(Promote warmth, relaxation, and kidney support)

- Ginger tea, cinnamon tea, chai
- Miso soup, barley tea, rooibos tea
- Herbal tonics with reishi, ashwagandha, or ginseng

WINTER EATING TIPS:

1. **Eat warm, cooked foods** to support digestion and maintain internal warmth.
2. **Include more warming herbs and spices** to enhance circulation and strengthen immunity.
3. **Reduce cold, raw, and excessive dairy** as they can weaken digestion and create internal dampness.
4. **Prioritize deeply nourishing, slow-cooked meals** like stews, soups, and broths to support kidney essence.

By following TCM's seasonal wisdom, you can replenish your energy, support kidney health, and fortify your body for winter's colder, introspective months.

NOURISHING THE WATER ELEMENT: YOGA, PRANAYAMA, MEDITATION, AND AROMATHERAPY FOR WINTER

In yoga, the Water element represents fluidity, introspection, and stillness. It governs the Kidneys and Urinary Bladder meridians in Chinese medicine, linking us to our deep reserves of energy, vitality, and emotional resilience. During the winter season, which is aligned with the Water element, it is important to support the kidneys, balance the flow of energy, and nurture a deep sense of inner calm.

Yoga, pranayama, meditation, and aromatherapy offer powerful tools for nourishing the Water element within the body and mind. Through forward bends, hip openers, and gentle, grounding flows, we can release tension and create space for a free flow of energy.

Yin yoga, known for its long-held stretches and deep relaxation, is especially beneficial for nourishing the Water element. This style of practice encourages stillness and introspection, helping us access the depths of our inner world and connect with the quieter rhythms of life.

Here are some key poses to incorporate into your practice:

<u>Butterfly Pose (Baddha Konasana)</u>

How to practice:

1. Sit on the floor with your spine tall and bring the soles of your feet together, allowing your knees to fall outward.
2. Hold onto your feet or ankles, keeping your chest open and shoulders relaxed.
3. For a dynamic variation, gently flutter your knees up and down like butterfly wings to encourage circulation.
4. For a deeper stretch, hinge at the hips and fold forward over your feet, keeping your spine long.
5. Stay in the pose for 30 seconds to a minute, breathing deeply into the stretch.

Benefits:

- Opens the hips, groin, and inner thighs, areas that hold tension and stagnation in winter.
- Stimulates Kidney 1 (Bubbling Spring) at the soles of the feet, promoting grounding and circulation.
- Encourages fluidity, flexibility, and emotional release.

<u>Chair Pose (Utkatasana)</u>

How to practice:

1. Stand with your feet together or hip-width apart, arms at your sides.

2. Inhale, then as you exhale, bend your knees, lowering your hips as if you're sitting in an imaginary chair.
3. Keep your weight in your heels and your chest lifted, arms reaching overhead.
4. Engage your core and lower back, drawing strength from the Kidney meridian.
5. Hold for 5–10 deep breaths, then slowly return to standing.

Benefits:

- Builds endurance, inner heat, and strength, counteracting winter's cold.
- Grounds and stabilizes energy, supporting the Kidneys.
- Boosts circulation and ignites Agni (digestive fire), reducing winter stagnation.

Modification: Add Ujjayi breath for extra warmth, or follow with a gentle forward fold to release tension.

Easy Sphinx Pose (Saral Bhujangasana)

How to practice:

1. Lie face down with your legs extended, elbows under your shoulders.
2. Press forearms into the floor as you gently lift your chest, opening the heart.
3. Keep your shoulders relaxed and spine long, breathing deeply into your lower back.
4. Hold for 5–10 breaths, feeling the Kidney meridian activate in the lower belly, inner legs and groin region.Encourages circulation and warmth in the lower back and Kidneys.

Benefits:

- Gently stretches the spine and chest, supporting a feeling of nourishment and vitality.

- Helps combat winter lethargy with slow, mindful breathing.

Hare Pose/Child's Pose (Shashankasana)

How to practice:

1. Kneel on the floor with your big toes touching, knees wide apart, buttocks moving toward the heels.
2. Fold forward, resting your forehead on the floor or mat and extend your arms forward or alongside your body.
3. Breathe deeply into your lower back and belly, allow the belly to release into the thighs and feel the tension release.
4. Hold for 30 seconds to 1 minute or longer, allowing complete relaxation.

Benefits:

- Activates the Kidney and Urinary Bladder meridians, promoting deep rest and restoration.
- Releases tension and tightness from the back and hips.
- Encourages introspection and stillness, aligning with the reflective energy of winter.

Mountain Pose/Downward Facing Dog (Parvatasana)

How to practice:

1. Start in a tabletop position, hands under shoulders, knees under hips.
2. Tuck your toes under and lift your hips toward the ceiling, straightening your legs.
3. Keep your hands firmly pressed into the mat, shoulders relaxed, and heels reaching toward the ground. Head aligned between shoulders.
4. Breathe deeply for 5–10 breaths, focusing on lengthening the spine and warming the body.

Benefits:

- Stimulates the Urinary Bladder meridian, releasing stagnation from the back body.
- Generates inner heat, essential for winter's slower metabolism.
- Strengthens the nervous system, helping to regulate stress and winter blues.
- Modification: Slightly bend the knees to ease tension and focus on steady, warming breaths.

PRANAYAMA (BREATHING TECHNIQUES) FOR WINTER

Pranayama techniques that focus on slow, deep breathing and balancing the body's energy are essential for nourishing the Kidneys and promoting emotional stability during winter. These practices can help soothe the mind, enhance vitality, and support the harmonious flow of energy through the Water element.

Ujjayi Pranayama (Victorious Breath)

Ujjayi Pranayama is a slow, controlled breath that creates a gentle oceanic sound in the back of the throat. It promotes focus, deep relaxation, and inner warmth, making it a wonderful breath practice to incorporate into asana practice or meditation.

How to Practice:

1. Find a comfortable seat or lie down. Sit in a relaxed but upright position, or rest in a supine pose like Savasana.
2. Close your mouth and breathe through your nose. Begin by inhaling and exhaling naturally.
3. Slightly constrict the back of your throat. As you breathe in and out through your nose, gently contract the muscles at the back of your throat, creating a soft whispering sound, similar to ocean waves or distant wind. Or you might imagine gently sipping through a straw in the same area.

4. Maintain a steady rhythm. Keep your inhales and exhales equal in length, ensuring smooth and steady breathing.
5. Deepen your breath. Expand your belly on the inhale and draw your navel slightly in on the exhale.
6. Continue for 5–10 minutes. If practicing during yoga, maintain Ujjayi breath throughout your asana flow.

Benefits:

- Promotes relaxation and mental clarity
- Warms the body and supports circulation
- Encourages deep focus during yoga or meditation
- Helps regulate the nervous system

Anuloma Viloma (Alternate-Nostril Breathing)

Anuloma Viloma, a variation of Nadi Shodhana Pranayama, is a balancing breath that helps generate inner warmth, calm the mind, and support the body's resilience during colder months. By briefly retaining the breath, the practice builds internal heat, supporting circulation and enhancing mental stillness.

How to Practice:

1. Find a comfortable seat. Sit in a relaxed, upright position with a straight spine.
2. Use Nasagra Mudra with your right hand (Rest the index and middle fingers on the eyebrow center. Relax your hand.) Use your right thumb to close your right nostril. Use your ring finger to close your left nostril.
3. Close the right nostril with your thumb and breathe in deeply through the left nostril.
4. Hold the breath for a few counts. Close both nostrils and retain the breath for 4–10 heartbeats. Keep this gentle and comfortable.
5. Exhale through the right nostril. Release your ring finger and exhale slowly through the right nostril.

6. Inhale through the right nostril. With the left nostril still open, take a slow and steady inhale.
7. Hold the breath again. Close both nostrils and hold for a few heartbeats.
8. Exhale through the left nostril. Release the right nostril and exhale smoothly.
9. Repeat for 5–10 minutes. Continue this cycle, alternating nostrils after each breath.

Tips:

- Keep the breath retention short and comfortable to avoid strain.
- Maintain a steady rhythm, ensuring inhales and exhales are even in length.
- Focus on deep, smooth breathing to calm the mind and promote warmth.

Benefits:

- Generates internal heat and enhances circulation
- Balances the nervous system and relieves stress
- Clears the mind, improving focus and clarity
- Supports the Water element and Kidney energy in Traditional Chinese Medicine, which governs resilience and deep reserves of energy

By incorporating Ujjayi Pranayama and Anuloma Viloma into your winter routine, you can cultivate warmth, steadiness, and mental clarity, aligning with the season's introspective and restorative energy.

MEDITATIONS FOR THE WATER ELEMENT: CULTIVATING STILLNESS AND INNER WISDOM

Meditation practices that focus on the Kidneys and Water element can help deepen our connection to our inner selves, promote emotional resilience, and access the quiet wisdom within. These practices support the flow of Qi (life force) and create space for reflection and renewal.

Kidney Meditation

This meditation is designed to strengthen and nourish the Kidney energy, which governs vitality, willpower, and deep reserves of energy in Traditional Chinese Medicine (TCM). The Kidneys are considered the storehouse of Jing (essence), making this practice ideal for restoring energy, resilience, and inner peace.

How to Practice:

1. Find a comfortable seated position. Sit in a cross-legged position, in a chair with feet flat on the floor, or in a gentle reclined position if preferred. Keep your spine straight and shoulders relaxed.
2. Close your eyes and focus on your lower back. Bring your awareness to the area just above your waist, on either side of your spine—where the kidneys are located.
3. Visualize a dark blue or deep indigo light. Imagine this light gently surrounding your kidneys, providing warmth, strength, and nourishment.
4. Breathe deeply. With each inhale, visualize the blue light expanding, infusing your kidneys with vitality. With each exhale, release any tension or fear stored in this area.
5. Affirm resilience and stability. Silently repeat a simple affirmation, such as *"My energy is strong and resilient"* or *"I am grounded, restored, and at peace."*
6. Continue for 5–10 minutes. Stay with this visualization, allowing the energy to build and bring a sense of balance and renewal.
7. Gently return to the present moment. Open your eyes and take a moment to notice how you feel.

Benefits:

- Strengthens the Kidney energy, supporting endurance and resilience
- Helps relieve fatigue, anxiety, and fear
- Encourages a deep sense of grounding and inner stillness
- Supports overall vitality, especially in winter or times of depletion

Water Element Visualization

This guided visualization connects you to the Water element, which represents flow, adaptability, and emotional depth. It is particularly beneficial for reducing stress, promoting inner peace, and cultivating a sense of renewal.

How to Practice:

1. Find a quiet place to sit or lie down. Make sure you are comfortable and free from distractions. Close your eyes and take a few deep breaths to settle in.
2. Visualize a body of water. Imagine yourself beside a tranquil lake, a flowing river, or the vast, rhythmic ocean. Choose an image that feels deeply calming and inviting to you.
3. Feel the movement of the water. Picture gentle ripples or waves moving in harmony, symbolizing the natural cycles of life. Imagine the soothing sound of water flowing, filling the space around you with peace.
4. Let the water cleanse and refresh you. With each inhale, imagine the water's energy washing over you, absorbing tension and stress. With each exhale, release any heaviness or stagnation, allowing it to dissolve into the currents.
5. Embrace fluidity and ease. Silently repeat an affirmation, such as *"I flow effortlessly with life"* or *"I am calm, clear, and deeply refreshed."*
6. Stay in this visualization for 5–10 minutes. Allow yourself to fully immerse in the experience, feeling a deep sense of relaxation and connection to the Water element.

7. Slowly return to the present moment. Bring your awareness back to your body, gently open your eyes, and take a few grounding breaths before resuming your day.

Benefits:

- Encourages emotional release and relaxation
- Reduces stress and mental clutter
- Aligns with the Water element's qualities of renewal, intuition, and fluidity
- Promotes adaptability and ease in times of change

Both Kidney Meditation and Water Element Visualization are powerful practices for harmonizing the body's energy, especially during winter or periods of emotional or physical depletion. These techniques help cultivate inner strength, adaptability, and deep restoration, fostering balance in both body and mind.

QIGONG FOR WINTER: CULTIVATING WARMTH AND LONGEVITY

"Kidney Warming Flow" (Water Element – Kidneys & Bladder)

Purpose: This practice supports the Kidney meridian, which stores our energy reserves, helping to cultivate warmth and longevity.

How to Practice:

1. Stand with Feet Together & Hands on the Lower Back – Press palms gently on the kidney area (just above the waistline).
2. Inhale & Rub Hands in Circles – Warm the lower back with gentle circular rubbing motions.
3. Exhale & Bend Slightly Forward – Allow a natural stretch in the spine, feeling warmth spreading through the back.
4. Inhale & Straighten Up – Continue to rub the kidney area, imagining deep reserves of energy being replenished.

5. Repeat for 2–3 minutes, breathing slowly and deeply.
6. Visualize a warm blue light surrounding the kidneys, like a deep ocean of stillness and energy reserves.

SENSORY ACTIVITIES

Sight: Witness the Tranquil Beauty of Winter Landscapes

Snowy Scenery Photography: Take a walk through a winter wonderland where snow blankets the earth and transforms the landscape into a peaceful scene of white. Capture the beauty of snow-covered trees, frosted branches, and the soft play of light on icy surfaces. Whether using a camera or simply enjoying the view, take time to appreciate the simplicity and purity of winter's natural beauty.

Stargazing on Clear Winter Nights: Winter skies are often crisp and clear, offering the perfect opportunity to gaze at the stars. Spend an evening stargazing, allowing the vastness of the night sky to ground you in the present moment. The shimmering constellations and the peaceful stillness of winter nights can evoke a sense of wonder and connection to the universe.

Sound: Tune into the Subtle Rhythms of Winter

Fireplace Crackling: There is something deeply soothing about the sound of a fireplace crackling, especially during the colder months. The gentle pop and hiss of burning wood, along with the warmth it radiates, creates a cozy atmosphere. Spend time relaxing near the fire, listening to the rhythmic sounds as you reflect, or enjoy a quiet moment of peace.

The Silence of Snowfall: When snow falls, it brings with it a profound silence—a quiet that blankets everything in its path. Walk through the snow, allowing the gentle crunch beneath your boots to bring you into a deep state of mindfulness. The stillness of snow offers an opportunity for introspection and presence, allowing you to hear the subtle sounds of nature in a way that is often missed during busier seasons.

Taste: Indulge in Winter's Comforting Flavors

Hot Cocoa Indulgence: Treat yourself to a comforting mug of hot cocoa (or raw cacao) topped as you choose. Savor the rich, chocolaty flavor and warmth it brings. Hot drinks like cocoa, herbal teas, and spiced cider are perfect for winter, as they not only nourish the body but also help you slow down and enjoy the cozy atmosphere of the season.

Hearty Winter Meals: Winter is a time to enjoy hearty, warming foods that provide comfort and nourishment. Experiment with root vegetables like sweet potatoes, carrots, and parsnips, or create rich, flavorful stews using seasonal ingredients. Cook meals that nourish both your body and your soul—whether it's a slow-cooked soup, a warm pie, or roasted vegetables, the flavors of winter offer a grounding experience.

Smell: Immerse Yourself in the Fragrances of Winter

Baking Session: Spend an afternoon baking cookies, pies, or bread. The aroma of freshly baked goods filling the air is one of winter's most comforting sensory experiences. Infuse your home with the scents of cinnamon, nutmeg, and vanilla, evoking feelings of warmth and nostalgia. This sensory activity can bring you closer to the essence of winter—nurturing, nourishing, and cozy.

Outdoor Scents of Winter: Take time to inhale the crisp, clean scent of fresh snow and pine trees during outdoor winter adventures. Whether walking in the woods, hiking in the mountains, or simply taking a stroll in the park, the earthy aroma of winter's forest and the freshness of snow provide an invigorating contrast to the warmth of home.

Touch: Ground Yourself in Winter's Sensations

Snowball Fight: Bundle up in warm layers and engage in a playful snowball fight with friends or family. Feel the cold snow against your gloves, the texture of fresh powder, and the exhilaration of the cold air on your skin. The physical activity of a snowball fight not only stimulates the body but also connects you to the playful energy of winter.

Cozy Blanket Snuggle: Winter is the perfect time to relax indoors, wrapping yourself in a warm, soft blanket. Snuggle up with a cup of hot beverage, a good book, or simply enjoy the peaceful quiet outside. The feeling of being swathed in warmth while the world outside is cold creates a perfect cocoon of comfort and security.

AROMATHERAPY FOR WINTER: ESSENTIAL OILS TO SUPPORT THE WATER ELEMENT

Aromatherapy offers a natural way to support the Water element during the winter months. Essential oils with calming, grounding, and respiratory support properties can help nourish the Kidneys, promote relaxation, and foster immune system health.

Here are some essential oils that align with the energy of the Water element:

1. Eucalyptus

Eucalyptus oil helps **clear congestion** and promotes **respiratory health**, making it perfect for winter. It supports the **lungs** and can aid in clearing blocked energy, providing a sense of relief and rejuvenation.

2. Peppermint

Peppermint provides a **cooling** and invigorating sensation, helping to clear the sinuses and promote easier breathing. It helps stimulate the **Kidneys**, supports digestion, and clears mental fog.

3. Tea Tree

Tea Tree is **antimicrobial** and **immune-boosting**, ideal for supporting respiratory health and aiding in the prevention of common winter illnesses. It also has a soothing effect on the skin and supports overall health.

4. Lemon

Lemon oil is **uplifting** and **refreshing**, helping to boost your mood and energy levels. Its clean citrus scent promotes mental clarity and emotional rejuvenation, which is crucial during the winter season.

5. Lavender

Lavender oil is known for its **calming** and **soothing** properties. It promotes relaxation, reduces **stress** and **anxiety**, and supports overall emotional balance, making it an excellent choice for nurturing the **Water element**.

6. Rosemary

Rosemary oil is **invigorating** and **stimulating**, enhancing **mental clarity** and **focus**. It also supports **respiratory health** and can help clear the mind, making it ideal for both physical and emotional rejuvenation.

7. Cinnamon

Cinnamon oil has a **warming** and **comforting** aroma, promoting **circulation** and **digestive health**. It also creates a cozy, nurturing atmosphere, helping you stay grounded during the winter season.

8. Frankincense

Frankincense is deeply **grounding** and **calming**, promoting emotional well-being and reducing feelings of **anxiety** and **depression**. Its deep, resinous aroma encourages stillness, making it ideal for connecting with your inner wisdom.

9. Bergamot

Bergamot oil has an **uplifting** citrus aroma that combats **winter blues**, helps to reduce **stress**, and supports emotional balance, offering comfort and encouragement during the colder months.

10. Ginger

Ginger oil is **warming** and **invigorating**, aiding in digestion, boosting immunity, and alleviating **muscle aches** and **pains.** It helps invigorate the **Kidneys** and supports the flow of energy throughout the body.

USING ESSENTIAL OILS SAFELY

As with all essential oils, be sure to follow proper dilution and usage guidelines. When using citrus oils, such as Lemon and Bergamot, be cautious of photo sensitivity. Always consult a qualified aromatherapist or healthcare professional for personalized guidance, especially if you have specific health concerns.

*Refer to Part 3: Chapter 8- Smell, for more on the Safe usage of essential oils.

CONCLUSION: NURTURING THE WATER ELEMENT IN WINTER

Winter is a season that invites us to slow down, reflect, and replenish. By engaging the senses in the activities of the season—whether through savoring comforting flavors, basking in the warmth of a fire, or enjoying the peaceful sounds of nature—we can deepen our connection to winter's energy of stillness and renewal.

By embracing the Water element through nourishment, reflection, and introspection, we honor the rhythms of nature and cultivate a sense of inner peace. Through mindful practices, grounding foods, and self-care rituals, we can recharge our vital energy (Qi), preparing ourselves for the energetic burst of growth and renewal that comes with the arrival of spring.

Let winter's quiet beauty guide you toward inner strength, clarity, and resilience, allowing you to tap into the deep reserves of wisdom and potential that reside within.

PART IV
RECIPES & DIY AROMA CARE

Part Four is dedicated to seasonally inspired and delicious Nutritional recipes and DIY Aromatherapy blends, designed to support your well-being through mindful nutrition and aroma sensory healing.

This is where you'll find nourishment for your senses through seasonal nutrition and aromatherapy. Each season has its own set of nutrient-rich recipes and DIY aromatherapy blends to help support your health, mood, and energy.

Recipes align with the principles of Chinese Medicine and seasonal living, to help to strengthen your digestion, balance your energy, and promote overall vitality. Additionally, the aromatherapy recipes offer simple yet effective ways to integrate the therapeutic benefits of Essential oils into your home and body care routines.

18
YUMMY NUTRITIONAL RECIPES FOR EACH SEASON

SPRING RECIPES

Citrus Cleanser

Ingredients:

- Juice of 2 oranges
- Juice of 1 lemon
- Juice of 1 lime
- 4 cups cold water
- 2 tablespoons honey or maple syrup (adjust to taste)
- Ice cubes
- Fresh mint leaves for garnish (optional)

Directions:

1. Strain the citrus through a fine-mesh sieve to remove any seeds or pulp as desired.

2. In a pitcher, mix together the orange juice, lemon juice, lime juice, and cold water.
3. Stir in the honey or agave syrup, adjusting the sweetness to your preference.
4. Fill glasses with ice cubes.
5. Pour the citrus cleanser mixture over the ice, dividing it evenly between glasses.
6. Stir gently to combine the flavors.
7. Garnish with fresh mint leaves, if desired.
8. Serve immediately and enjoy the cool and refreshing flavors of citrus and mint in this spunky spring beverage.

This citrus cleanser is a delicious and hydrating drink that combines the natural sweetness of spring with the tangy and refreshing flavors of citrus fruits. It's perfect for starting to clear out our lymphatic systems after winters heavier diet and more sedentary lifestyle.

Nettle Pesto

Nettle is a tonic herb that is often used as a nourishing and tasty food, a strengthening and refreshing tea, a support for healthy urinary function with a mild diuretic action*, and as a mild astringent.

This pesto makes a tasty spread on bread or crackers, a delicious dip for fresh veggies, or a sauce for pasta. It keeps in the fridge for up to a month and freezes well too.

Ingredients:

- 2-4 Tbsp. organic hulled hemp seeds, pine nuts, walnuts, or other nut/seed of your choice
- 4-5 oz. fresh nettle leaves and stems (or 2 cups dried organic nettle leaf)
- 2-3 oz. grated organic Parmigiano Reggiano

- 1/2-1 tsp. finely ground sea salt or other salt of your choosing, or to taste
- 1-2 peeled organic garlic cloves (or 1-2 tsp. organic garlic powder), or to taste
- 3/4 cup organic extra virgin olive oil, or to desired consistency

Directions:

1. Bring a large pot of water to boil.
2. Set aside a large bowl of ice water.
3. Toast hemp seeds or other nut/seeds on a hot frying pan for about 1 minute, or until golden brown (but not burned). Remove from heat.
4. Once the water boils, place the nettle into boiling water using tongs. *If using a fresh nettle, be very careful not to touch it with your bare hands!
5. Blanch nettle for 1 to 2 minutes. This will remove the sting.
6. Remove the nettle from boiling water and place it in a bowl of ice water to help it retain its bright, green color.
7. Turn off the heat on boiling water. (reserve the water for boiling your pasta if you are using the pesto as a pasta sauce. It can also make for a nutritious tea!)
8. Once the nettle pulp has cooled (about 5 minutes) remove it by the handful and squeeze out most of the water.
9. Place squeezed nettle on a kitchen towel to dry.
10. Combine the nettle and remaining ingredients (except olive oil) in a food processor or blender.
11. Blend until ingredients are well mixed and form a paste.
12. With the blender or food processor running, slowly pour in oil until the desired consistency is reached.

Your pesto is now complete! Use immediately, refrigerate, or freeze. *Bon Appetit!*

Strawberry Basil Lemonade

Ingredients:

- 1 cup fresh strawberries, hulled and sliced
- Handful of fresh basil leaves
- Juice of 4-5 lemons
- 4 cups water
- 1/4 cup honey or maple syrup (adjust to taste)
- Ice cubes

Directions:

1. In a blender or food processor, blend the strawberries and basil leaves until smooth.
2. Strain the strawberry and basil mixture through a fine-mesh sieve to remove any solids.
3. In a pitcher, combine the strawberry-basil juice, lemon juice, water, and honey or maple syrup. Stir well to dissolve the sweetener.
4. Taste and adjust the sweetness or tartness by adding more honey/maple syrup or lemon juice, if desired.
5. Fill glasses with ice cubes.
6. Pour the strawberry basil lemonade over the ice cubes, dividing it evenly between glasses.
7. Stir gently to mix the flavors.
8. Garnish with a fresh strawberry or basil leaf, if desired.
9. Serve immediately and enjoy the refreshing combination of sweet strawberries, aromatic basil, and tangy lemon in this delightful spring beverage.

This strawberry basil lemonade is a perfect way to enjoy the juicy, bright flavors of summer.

The combination of ripe strawberries and fragrant basil adds a unique twist to traditional lemonade, making it more hydrating and a refreshing drink for the season.

Summer watermelon cucumber salad

Ingredients:

- 4 cups cubed watermelon
- 2 cups sliced cucumbers
- 1/4 cup fresh mint leaves, chopped
- 1/4 cup crumbled feta cheese (optional)
- Juice of 1 lime
- 1 tablespoon extra-virgin olive oil
- Salt and pepper to taste

Directions:

1. In a large bowl, combine the cubed watermelon, sliced cucumbers, and chopped mint leaves.
2. If using, sprinkle the crumbled feta cheese over the salad.
3. In a small bowl, whisk together the lime juice, olive oil, salt, and pepper.
4. Drizzle the dressing over the salad and gently toss to combine.
5. Let the salad sit for a few minutes to allow the flavors to meld together.
6. Serve the watermelon cucumber salad chilled and enjoy it as a refreshing side dish or light meal during the summer.

This salad is not only hydrating but also packed with vitamins and minerals from the watermelon and cucumbers. It's a perfect way to cool down and enjoy the flavors of summer!

Chia pudding for heart health

Ingredients:

- 2 tablespoons chia seeds
- 1 cup unsweetened almond milk (or any other plant-based milk)
- 1 tablespoon pure maple syrup (or sweetener of your choice)
- 1/2 teaspoon pure vanilla extract
- 1/2 cup mixed fresh berries (such as blueberries, raspberries, or strawberries)
- A handful of chopped nuts (such as walnuts or almonds) for added heart-healthy fats
- Fresh mint leaves for garnish (optional)

Directions:

1. In a bowl or jar, combine the chia seeds, almond milk, maple syrup, and vanilla extract. Stir well to ensure the chia seeds are evenly distributed.
2. Let the mixture sit for about 5 minutes, and then stir again to prevent clumping.
3. Cover the bowl or jar and refrigerate for at least 2 hours or overnight, allowing the chia seeds to absorb the liquid and thicken into a pudding-like consistency.
4. Once the chia pudding has set, give it a good stir to break up any clumps.
5. Layer the chia pudding with the mixed berries in serving glasses or bowls.
6. Top with chopped nuts for added texture and heart-healthy fats.
7. Garnish with fresh mint leaves if a little more cooling effect is desired.

LATE SUMMER RECIPES

Delicious Date Beverage

Ingredients:

- 10 dates, pitted and soaked in warm water for 15 minutes
- 2 cups coconut water
- 1 cup almond milk (or any plant-based milk of your choice)
- 1 teaspoon vanilla extract
- Ice cubes
- Optional: a pinch of ground cinnamon or nutmeg for added flavor

Directions:

1. Drain the soaked dates and discard the soaking water.
2. In a blender, combine the soaked dates, coconut water, almond milk, vanilla extract, and optional ground cinnamon or nutmeg.
3. Blend on high speed until the mixture is smooth and well combined.
4. Taste the beverage and adjust the sweetness or flavors as desired by adding more dates or spices.
5. Fill glasses with ice cubes.
6. Pour the date beverage over the ice, dividing it evenly between glasses.
7. Stir gently to chill the drink and incorporate the flavors.
8. Serve immediately and enjoy the creamy and naturally sweet taste of the date beverage.

This date beverage is perfect for late summer as dates are in season and provide a natural sweetness to the drink. Dates are also known for their nutritional benefits, including being a good source of fiber, vitamins, and minerals. The combination of coconut water and almond milk adds a creamy and refreshing element, while the hint of vanilla extract enhances the flavor profile. Sip and savor this delightful date beverage as a nourishing and hydrating treat during the late summer days.

Roasted Sweet Potato and Avocado Salad

Ingredients:

- 2 medium sweet potatoes, peeled and cubed
- 1 tablespoon olive oil
- 1 teaspoon paprika
- Salt and pepper to taste
- 2 cups mixed salad greens
- 1 ripe avocado, diced
- 1/4 cup cherry tomatoes, halved
- 1/4 cup crumbled feta cheese (optional)
- 2 tablespoons chopped fresh cilantro

For the dressing:

- 2 tablespoons olive oil
- 1 tablespoon lemon juice
- 1 teaspoon honey
- Salt and pepper to taste

Directions:

1. Preheat your oven to 400°F (200°C).
2. In a bowl, toss the sweet potato cubes with olive oil, paprika, salt, and pepper until well coated.
3. Spread the sweet potatoes in a single layer on a baking sheet lined with parchment paper. Roast for about 25-30 minutes

or until they are tender and slightly caramelized. Set aside to cool.

4. In a large salad bowl, combine the mixed salad greens, diced avocado, cherry tomatoes, and crumbled feta cheese (if using).
5. In a small bowl, whisk together the olive oil, lemon juice, honey, salt, and pepper to make the dressing.
6. Add the roasted sweet potatoes to the salad bowl and drizzle the dressing over the salad. Gently toss to combine.
7. Sprinkle the chopped cilantro over the top for garnish.

Serve the salad immediately and enjoy the flavors of late summer!

This salad is not only tasty but also packed with nutrients from sweet potatoes, avocado, and fresh vegetables. It's a perfect light and refreshing dish to savor during the late summer season.

AUTUMN RECIPES

Fall Spiced Apple Cider

Ingredients:

- 4 cups apple cider
- 2 cups water
- 2 cinnamon sticks
- 4 whole cloves
- 4 whole allspice berries
- 1 orange, sliced
- Optional: honey or maple syrup to sweeten (adjust to taste)

Directions:

1. In a large pot, combine the apple cider, water, cinnamon sticks, cloves, allspice berries, and orange slices.

2. Place the pot over medium heat and bring the mixture to a simmer. Let it simmer for about 20-30 minutes to allow the flavors to meld together.
3. Taste the cider, and if desired, sweeten with honey or maple syrup to your liking. Stir well to dissolve the sweetener.
4. Remove the pot from heat and strain the cider to remove the spices and orange slices.
5. Serve the warm spiced apple cider in mugs or cups.
6. Optionally, garnish each serving with a fresh cinnamon stick or a slice of orange.

Enjoy the cozy and comforting flavors of fall with this spiced apple cider. The combination of cinnamon, cloves, and allspice infuses the cider with warm and aromatic notes. The orange slices add a touch of brightness to the drink. Sip on this delightful beverage during chilly autumn days, whether you're gathered around a bonfire, enjoying a relaxing evening at home, or hosting a festive gathering.

Shitake Quinoa Salad

Ingredients:

- 1 cup uncooked quinoa
- 1 1/4 cups vegetable broth
- neutral oil, such as rice bran oil
- 3-4 shiitake mushrooms, sliced
- 1 shallot, thinly sliced
- 2-3 cups spinach (or greens of your choice)
- 1 avocado, sliced
- salt and freshly ground pepper
- sliced green onions to garnish

Dressing:

- 1 tablespoon finely chopped onion
- 2 tablespoons oil of choice (olive, avocado...)
- 1 tablespoon soy sauce
- 2 tablespoons rice vinegar
- 1 teaspoon brown sugar
- 1/2 lemon juice

Directions:

1. Start off by cooking the quinoa. If you have your tried and true method of cooking quinoa that works for you, ignore this next little bit. Rinse quinoa in a fine mesh strainer and then drain well. Sometimes, I cook my quinoa in my rice cooker, but if I'm doing it in a pot, I use a non-stick one. Add the drained quinoa to your non-stick pot and turn the heat to medium to slightly toast the kernels for about 2 minutes.
2. Add the 1 1/4 cups of broth, bring to a boil, turn the heat down to low and cover.
3. Cook for 15 minutes. Then remove the pot from the burner and let the quinoa sit, covered, for 5 minutes.
4. After 5 minutes, lift the lid and fluff.
5. Let the quinoa cool while you're preparing the other ingredients.
6. Heat up oil in a non-stick skillet or a cast iron pan over medium heat.
7. Add the mushroom slices in a single layer and cook undisturbed until golden and crispy, about 2-3 minutes.
8. Flip and continue to cook. Cook until the mushrooms should be slightly shriveled and golden in color. Drain on paper towels and repeat until all of the mushroom slices are cooked. Season the mushrooms with salt and pepper while still hot.
9. Add two and a half tablespoons of oil to the same skillet and heat over medium-low heat. Add the sliced shallots and

gently fry, stirring occasionally, until they turn golden brown, about 5-8 minutes. Keep a close watch, as shallots can deepen in color quite quickly. When golden, turn off the heat, scoop out the shallots, and drain on paper towels. Let the shallot oil cool and set aside for the dressing.

10. In the same skillet, quickly wilt the spinach (or greens of choice). Season with salt and pepper and set aside. Whisk together the dressing ingredients and toss into the quinoa. I use all of the dressing, but start out with half and taste as you go. To plate, scoop a generous amount of quinoa on a plate or in a bowl. Top with the mushrooms, greens, and sliced avocado. Garnish with the crispy shallots and green onions. Enjoy!

WINTER RECIPES

Black Sesame Candy

Ingredients:

- 1 cup black sesame seeds
- 1 cup honey
- 1/4 cup sugar
- 1 tablespoon butter
- Optional: toasted sesame seeds for coating

Directions:

1. In a dry pan, toast the black sesame seeds over medium heat until fragrant. Let them cool.
2. Grind the toasted black sesame seeds in a blender or food processor until finely ground. Set aside.
3. In a saucepan, combine the honey, sugar, and butter. Heat

over medium-low heat, stirring continuously, until the sugar has dissolved and the mixture is well combined.

4. Add the ground black sesame seeds to the saucepan and mix thoroughly.
5. Continue cooking the mixture over medium-low heat, stirring constantly, until it thickens and starts to pull away from the sides of the pan. This usually takes about 10-15 minutes.
6. Once the mixture has thickened, remove it from the heat and let it cool slightly.
7. Grease a baking dish or line it with parchment paper. Pour the black sesame mixture into the dish and spread it evenly.
8. Let the mixture cool completely and set, either at room temperature or in the refrigerator.
9. Once fully cooled and set, cut the black sesame mixture into small squares or rectangles.
10. Optional: Roll the cut pieces in toasted sesame seeds for an extra layer of flavor and texture.

Store the black sesame candy in an airtight container at room temperature.

These black sesame candies are a delicious and nutritious treat. The rich, nutty flavor of the black sesame seeds combined with the sweetness of honey and sugar creates a delightful candy that can be enjoyed anytime. It's a great snack to satisfy your sweet tooth while also incorporating the goodness of black sesame seeds.

**In Traditional Chinese Medicine (TCM), black sesame seeds are believed to have several medicinal properties that can nourish the kidneys and support overall health. Black sesame seeds are considered a tonic for the kidneys, which are associated with vital energy and longevity in TCM. They are also believed to nourish the blood and yin, improve digestion, and promote healthy hair growth. Black sesame helps promote healthy, lustrous hair and even darken prematurely gray hair.

Cardamom green tea latte

**This is Erika's signature beverage of choice! An adaptation from Kashmiri Green tea, which she got hooked on in Kashmir, India, during a trek in the Himalayas several decades ago. More on that story another time!

Ingredients:

- 1 cup milk (such as raw cow, almond milk, oat milk, or coconut milk)
- 1 teaspoon matcha green tea powder (or regular green tea works too)
- 1/2 teaspoon ground cardamom (or one drop of cardamom EO vitality)
- Sweetener of choice (such as raw stevia, maple syrup or honey)
- Optional: a dash of vanilla extract

Instructions:

1. In a small saucepan, heat the non-dairy milk over medium heat until hot but not boiling. Remove from heat.
2. In a separate bowl, whisk together the matcha green tea powder, ground cardamom, sweetener, and vanilla extract (if using) until well combined.
3. Slowly pour the hot, non-dairy milk into the matcha mixture while whisking continuously to create a frothy texture.
4. Once well combined and frothy, pour the latte into a mug and serve hot.
5. Optionally, you can sprinkle a pinch of ground cardamom on top for added flavor and presentation.

Note: Adjust the amount of sweetener according to your taste preferences. You can also adjust the ratio of matcha powder/green tea and cardamom based on your desired strength of flavors. Feel free to experiment and make it just right for you!

Cardamom, an aromatic spice native to India, has been widely used for centuries in traditional medicine practices such as Ayurveda and traditional Chinese medicine.

It possesses various medicinal properties that contribute to its potential health benefits including the following:

1. **Digestive Health:** Cardamom is known for its carminative properties, which can help alleviate digestive issues such as indigestion, bloating, and flatulence. It may promote the secretion of digestive enzymes and enhance the absorption of nutrients, supporting overall digestive health.
2. **Anti-inflammatory Effects:** Cardamom contains compounds with anti-inflammatory properties, such as cineole and alpha-terpinyl acetate. These compounds have been found to help reduce inflammation in the body, potentially benefiting conditions like arthritis and inflammatory diseases.
3. **Antimicrobial Properties:** The essential oils present in cardamom, such as terpinen-4-ol and linalool, possess antimicrobial properties. These properties may help combat bacteria, viruses, and fungi, contributing to better oral health and potentially reducing the risk of infections.
4. **Antioxidant Activity:** Cardamom is rich in antioxidants, such as flavonoids and phenolic compounds. These antioxidants help protect the body against oxidative stress caused by free radicals, which can contribute to various chronic diseases and premature aging.
5. **Respiratory Health:** The aromatic properties of cardamom make it beneficial for respiratory health. It may help relieve congestion, coughs, and respiratory conditions like bronchitis and asthma by promoting expectoration and opening up the airways.

6. **Blood Pressure and Heart Health:** Some studies suggest that cardamom may help lower blood pressure levels, potentially reducing the risk of cardiovascular diseases. It may also help improve lipid profiles by reducing LDL cholesterol and triglyceride levels.

Root Soup

A nourishing and grounding recipe to warm you from the inside out! Also one of Erika's favorite dishes for the season.

Ingredients:

- 1 large beet (1/2 pound)—peeled, halved and sliced 1/3 inch thick
- 1 medium turnip (1/2 pound)—peeled, halved and sliced 1/3 inch thick
- 1 medium parsnip (1/2 pound)—peeled and sliced on the diagonal 1/3 inch thick
- 1 medium onion, thickly sliced
- 2 tablespoons extra-virgin olive oil
- 4 cups chicken or veg stock or any low-sodium broth
- Salt and freshly ground pepper
- Crème fraîche or sour cream, for serving
- 1 1/2 tablespoons chopped fresh dill

Directions:

1. Preheat the oven to 500°. On a large-rimmed baking sheet, toss the beet, turnip, parsnip, and onion with the olive oil and spread in a single layer.
2. Roast the vegetables for about 20 minutes, stirring once or twice, until tender and golden brown around the edges.
3. Transfer the vegetables to a large saucepan.
4. Add the stock, cover, and bring to a boil.

5. Simmer over low heat until the vegetables are tender, about 10 minutes.
6. Working in batches, puree the soup in a blender or food processor until smooth. (Alternatively, use an immersion blender to puree the soup.)
7. Return the soup to the saucepan and reheat gently.
8. Season with salt and pepper.
9. Ladle the soup into deep bowls.
10. Top with a dollop of crème fraîche and the chopped fresh dill, and serve at once. Enjoy!

Magical Mineral Broth

"This rejuvenating liquid, rich in magnesium, potassium, and sodium, helps the body refresh and restore itself. I think of it as a tonic, designed to keep you in top form. It serves as everything from a delicious sipping tea to a powerful base for hearty soups and stews. No matter one's appetite, it provides a tremendous nutritional boost." *From* Cancer Fighting Kitchen by Rebecca Katz

Ingredients:

- 6 unpeeled carrots, cut into thirds
- 2 unpeeled yellow onions, cut into chunks
- 1 leek, white and green parts, cut into thirds
- 1 bunch celery, including the heart, cut into thirds
- 4 unpeeled red potatoes, quartered
- 2 unpeeled Japanese or regular sweet potatoes, quartered
- 1 unpeeled garnet yam, quartered
- 5 unpeeled cloves garlic, halved
- 1/2 bunch fresh flat-leaf parsley
- 1 8-inch strip of kombu seaweed
- a few black peppercorns
- 4 whole allspice or juniper berries
- 2 bay leaves

- 8 quarts cold, filtered water
- 1 teaspoon sea salt

Instructions:

1. Rinse all of the vegetables well, including the kombu. In a 12-quart or larger stockpot, combine the carrots, onions, leek, celery, potatoes, sweet potatoes, yam, garlic, parsley, kombu, peppercorns, allspice berries, and bay leaves. Fill the pot with the water to 2 inches below the rim, cover, and bring to a boil.
2. Remove the lid, decrease the heat to low, and simmer, uncovered, for at least 2 hours. As the broth simmers, some of the water will evaporate; add more if the vegetables begin to peek out. Simmer until the full richness of the vegetables can be tasted.
3. Strain the broth through a large, coarse-mesh sieve (remember to use a heat-resistant container underneath), then add salt to taste. Let cool to room temperature before refrigerating or freezing.

COOK'S NOTE: Like fine wine, this broth gets better with age. The longer the simmer time, the better tasting and more nutrient-dense the broth will be. You can also cut the recipe in half and make it in a slow cooker or a pressure cooker. Kombu is dark brown seaweed (kelp) that is dried and folded into sheets. It's used in Japanese cooking to add depth and flavor to soups and stocks. It also adds a tremendous amount of valuable trace minerals to this broth. Look for kombu in the Asian section of many grocery stores or online.

STORAGE: Store in an airtight container in the refrigerator for 5 to 7 days or in the freezer for 4 months.

From Cancer Fighting Kitchen by Rebecca Katz

19
DO-IT-YOURSELF (DIY) AROMATHERAPY RECIPES

SPRING DIY

Spring cleansing spray

Ingredients:

- 10 drops of lemon essential oil
- 5 drops of grapefruit essential oil
- 3 drops of peppermint essential oil
- 2 drops of lavender essential oil
- 2 ounces of distilled water
- 1 ounce of witch hazel or vodka (as a dispersant)

Directions:

1. In a glass spray bottle, combine the distilled water and witch hazel/vodka.

2. Add the drops of lemon, grapefruit, peppermint, and lavender essential oils into the bottle.
3. Screw on the spray bottle cap and shake well to mix the ingredients thoroughly.

To use, simply shake the bottle before each use and spritz the cleansing blend in your space, such as your home, office, or car. You can also lightly mist it on linens or pillows for a fresh scent. As you do so, take deep breaths and envision the essential oils clearing away stagnant energy and promoting a sense of renewal and clarity. Citrus oils are uplifting and regenerative!

Remember to label your spray bottle and store it in a cool, dark place when not in use.

Diffuser Blend- The Allergy Trio

- 4 drops of Lavender
- 3 drops of Lemon
- 2 drops of Peppermint

Combine these essential oils in your diffuser with the recommended amount of water, and let the beautiful blend fill your space with the refreshing scents of spring. Adjust the number of drops according to your preference and the size of the room. Enjoy the rejuvenating and aromatic experience! Remember to follow safety guidelines for diffusing essential oils and ensure proper ventilation in the area.

SUMMER DIY

Peppermint Cooling Spray

- Drip 3-5 drops of therapeutic Peppermint essential oil in a 2 oz. Spray bottle.
- Fill the bottle with water
- Shake well, spritz on your chest, arms, feet, or neck, and COOL down!

This is definitely one of my Summer essentials and has a permanent place in my bag! You can add a drop of Lavender to soothe or a few drops of aloe vera gel for a little extra moisture.

Summer moisturizer

Ingredients:

- 1/4 cup shea butter
- 1/4 cup coconut oil
- 10 drops of lavender essential oil
- 8 drops of geranium essential oil
- 6 drops of ylang-ylang essential oil

Directions:

1. In a heat-safe bowl, melt the shea butter and coconut oil together using a double boiler or microwave in short bursts.
2. Once melted, remove it from the heat and let it cool slightly.
3. Add the lavender, geranium, and ylang-ylang essential oils to the mixture and stir well.
4. Transfer the mixture into a clean, airtight container, such as a glass jar or container.
5. Allow the moisturizer to solidify and cool completely before using.

To use, scoop a small amount of the moisturizer and gently massage it into your skin after cleansing. The combination of shea butter and coconut oil will provide hydration and nourishment, while the essential oils add a lovely aroma and potential benefits for your skin.

Remember to patch-test the moisturizer on a small area of your skin to check for any potential allergies or sensitivities before applying it to your face or body.

Diffuser Blend- Refresh and Enliven!

- 3 drops of Peppermint
- 3 drops of Sweet Orange
- 2 drops of Grapefruit
- 1 drop of Lemongrass

Combine these essential oils in a diffuser with the recommended amount of water and enjoy the invigorating and refreshing atmosphere in your space. Adjust the number of drops based on your personal preference and the size of the room. Remember to follow the safety guidelines for diffusing essential oils and ensure proper ventilation in the area.

After-sun cream

Ingredients:

- 1/4 cup aloe vera gel
- 2 tablespoons shea butter
- 1 tablespoon coconut oil
- 5 drops of lavender essential oil
- 3 drops peppermint essential oil
- 2 drops of chamomile essential oil

Directions:

1. In a double boiler or a heat-safe bowl, melt the shea butter and coconut oil over low heat until they are fully melted and combined.
2. Remove the mixture from heat and let it cool for a few minutes.
3. Add the aloe vera gel to the melted mixture and stir well until everything is thoroughly mixed.
4. Allow the mixture to cool completely before adding the essential oils to preserve their therapeutic properties.
5. Add the lavender, peppermint, and chamomile essential oils to the mixture and stir well.
6. Transfer the mixture into a clean, airtight container or jar.

Store the after-sun cream in a cool place and apply it generously to sun-exposed areas after sun exposure.

The soothing properties of aloe vera, combined with the moisturizing effects of shea butter and coconut oil, can help hydrate and nourish the skin after sun exposure. Lavender essential oil has calming and soothing properties, while peppermint essential oil provides a cooling sensation. Chamomile essential oil helps to reduce skin inflammation and promote skin healing.

Remember to do a patch test before using the cream on a larger area of your skin to ensure you don't have any sensitivities or allergies to the ingredients. If you experience any adverse reactions, discontinue use and consult a healthcare professional.

LATE SUMMER DIY

Grounding scrub for the Earth element

Ingredients:

- 1 cup of granulated sugar or sea salt

- 1/4 cup of carrier oil (such as sweet almond oil or coconut oil)
- 5 drops of patchouli essential oil
- 5 drops of vetiver essential oil
- 5 drops of cedarwood essential oil
- 5 drops of sandalwood essential oil
- 5 drops of frankincense essential oil

Directions:

1. In a mixing bowl, combine the granulated sugar or sea salt with the carrier oil.
2. Stir well until you achieve a consistent texture.
3. Add the essential oils (patchouli, vetiver, cedar wood, sandalwood, and frankincense) to the mixture.
4. Mix thoroughly to ensure that the essential oils are evenly distributed.
5. Transfer the scrub to a clean, airtight container for storage.
6. To use, take a small amount of the scrub and gently massage it onto damp skin in circular motions.
7. Rinse off with warm water and pat dry.
8. Enjoy the grounding and nurturing properties of the Earth element through the aromatic blend of essential oils in the scrub.

Perform a patch test before using the scrub on a larger area of your skin to ensure there are no sensitivities or allergies. Adjust the amount of carrier oil and essential oils according to your preference and the desired consistency of the scrub. Enjoy!

"Digestif" Blend

Ingredients:

- 4 drops of ginger essential oil

- 3 drops of peppermint essential oil
- 2 drops of fennel essential oil
- 2 drops of lemon essential oil
- 2 drops of chamomile essential oil
- 2 drops of patchouli essential oil

Directions:

1. In a small glass bottle or container, combine the drops of each essential oil.
2. Gently swirl or shake the bottle to mix the oils together.
3. To use, add a few drops of the blend to a carrier oil, such as fractionated coconut oil or jojoba oil, and massage onto your abdomen in a clockwise motion.
4. Alternatively, you can add a few drops of the blend to a diffuser and let the aroma fill the room while you relax.

Apply in a clockwise direction over the abdomen in the area of bloating or discomfort. Remember to perform a patch test before applying the blend to your skin and consult a healthcare professional if you have any specific health concerns or sensitivities.

AUTUMN DIY

Diffuser Blend-"Cozy Home"

Ingredients:

- 3 drops of cinnamon essential oil
- 3 drops of sweet orange essential oil
- 2 drops of clove essential oil
- 2 drops of ginger essential oil

Directions:

1. Fill your diffuser with water according to the manufacturer's instructions.
2. Add the specified number of drops of each essential oil to the water in the diffuser.
3. Turn on the diffuser and enjoy the aromatic blend as it fills the air.
4. Adjust the number of drops of each oil based on your personal preference and the size of your diffuser.
5. Feel free to experiment with the ratios or add other essential oils that evoke the cozy and warm feeling of autumn.

This blend combines the warm, spicy notes of cinnamon, clove, and ginger with the uplifting and refreshing scent of sweet orange. It creates a delightful and comforting ambiance in your home, bringing the essence of autumn indoors. Enjoy the cozy and inviting atmosphere that this seasonal diffuser blend creates during the autumn months.

Dry Nose and Immune Support roller

(or a dropper bottle works too!)

Ingredients:

- 1 tablespoon jojoba oil
- 2 drops eucalyptus essential oil
- 2 drops of tea tree essential oil
- 2 drops of lavender essential oil

Directions:

1. In a small, clean bottle or container, add the jojoba oil.
2. Add the eucalyptus essential oil, tea tree essential oil, and lavender essential oil to the jojoba oil.

3. Close the bottle or container and gently roll or shake to mix the oils together.

To use, apply a small amount of the blend to the fingertips and gently massage it around the nostrils. You can also inhale the aroma for respiratory support. The jojoba oil provides a moisturizing base, while the eucalyptus, tea tree, and lavender essential oils offer properties that can help soothe a dry nose and provide immune system support.

Remember to perform a patch test before applying the blend to your skin, especially if you have sensitive skin. Adjust the essential oil quantities based on your preference and personal sensitivity.

WINTER DIY

Warming Massage Oil

Ingredients:

- 3 drops of Ginger essential oil
- 3 drops of Cinnamon essential oil
- 2 drops of Sweet Orange essential oil
- 2 tablespoons of carrier oil (such as coconut or almond oil)

Directions:

Mix the essential oils with the carrier oil and use it for a soothing and warming massage to combat winter stiffness and promote relaxation. * Test a small area first to be sure the skin/body can tolerate it. Oils like cinnamon are considered 'hot" and need to be used mindfully. Add additional carrier oil to dilute as needed.

Comforting Bath Blend

Ingredients:

- 4 drops of Lavender essential oil
- 3 drops of Cedar wood essential oil
- 2 drops of Vetiver essential oil
- 1 cup of Epsom salt

Directions:

Mix the essential oils with Epsom salt and add it to a warm bath. Soak in the comforting aroma and let the oils relax your body and calm your mind.

Winter Room Spray

Ingredients:

- 10 drops of Pine essential oil
- 8 drops of Peppermint essential oil
- 6 drops of Juniper Berry essential oil
- Distilled water

Directions:

Combine the essential oils with distilled water in a spray bottle. Shake well before use and spritz it around your home to create a fresh and uplifting winter atmosphere.

***Remember to always follow safety guidelines and dilution ratios when using essential oils. Adjust the recipes according to your preferences and enjoy the benefits of these DIY blends during the winter season.

20
SEASONAL SHOPPING LISTS

SPRING SHOPPING LIST

- **Vegetables:** Leafy greens (spinach, kale, dandelion, arugula), sprouts, asparagus, artichokes, scallions, radishes
- **Fruits:** Citrus (lemon, grapefruit, oranges), apples, pears, cherries
- **Grains & Legumes:** Quinoa, brown rice, barley, lentils, mung beans
- **Herbs & Spices:** Milk thistle, turmeric, cilantro, parsley, rosemary, mint
- **Proteins:** Light fish, organic chicken, eggs, fermented foods (kimchi, miso, sauerkraut)
- **Essential Oils:** Lemon, rosemary, eucalyptus
- **Extras:** Green tea, apple cider vinegar, detoxifying herbal teas

SUMMER SHOPPING LIST

- **Vegetables:** Tomatoes, bell peppers, cucumbers, zucchini, summer squash, celery

- **Fruits:** Berries (strawberries, blueberries, raspberries), watermelon, mango, peaches
- **Grains & Legumes:** Amaranth, millet, chickpeas, sprouted grains
- **Herbs & Spices:** Basil, oregano, cilantro, cooling herbs (mint, dill)
- **Proteins:** Wild-caught fish, grass-fed meats, organic tofu, yogurt
- **Essential Oils:** Peppermint, lavender, jasmine
- **Extras:** Coconut water, aloe vera juice, hibiscus tea, cooling herbal teas

LATE SUMMER SHOPPING LIST

- **Vegetables:** Sweet potatoes, squash, carrots, beets, parsnips, yams
- **Fruits:** Peaches, plums, melons, figs, dates, papaya
- **Grains & Legumes:** Oats, quinoa, millet, chickpeas, lentils
- **Herbs & Spices:** Ginger, cinnamon, fennel, turmeric
- **Proteins:** Bone broth, tempeh, organic dairy, legumes
- **Essential Oils:** Ginger, chamomile, cardamom
- **Extras:** Herbal digestive teas, honey, golden milk

AUTUMN SHOPPING LIST

- **Vegetables:** Cabbage, cauliflower, daikon radish, leeks, garlic, onions
- **Fruits:** Apples, pears, persimmons, pomegranates, grapes
- **Grains & Legumes:** Brown rice, oats, white beans, adzuki beans
- **Herbs & Spices:** Mustard seed, horseradish, thyme, sage
- **Proteins:** Mushrooms, nuts (almonds, walnuts), eggs, tempeh
- **Essential Oils:** Frankincense, eucalyptus, pine
- **Extras:** White tea, ginger tea, herbal lung tonics

WINTER SHOPPING LIST

- **Vegetables:** Root vegetables (turnips, carrots, potatoes), dark leafy greens, seaweed, mushrooms
- **Fruits:** Dark berries, dried fruits (figs, dates), citrus
- **Grains & Legumes:** Black beans, kidney beans, wild rice, buckwheat
- **Herbs & Spices:** Garlic, black pepper, cinnamon, cloves, ginseng
- **Proteins:** Hearty broths, warming soups, fatty fish, grass-fed meats
- **Essential Oils:** Cedarwood, myrrh, vetiver
- **Extras:** Herbal adaptogens (ashwagandha, reishi), miso, warming teas

21
DIY SHOPPING LIST

DIY AROMATHERAPY SHOPPING LIST & TRUSTED SOURCES:

Stock up on these essential ingredients to create your own seasonal blends for relaxation, rejuvenation, and balance!

Base Ingredients (Use Year-Round)

Carrier Oils:

- Jojoba oil
- Sweet almond oil
- Coconut oil
- Olive oil
- Grapeseed oil
- Castor oil (for hair and digestive massage)

Essential Oil Blending Supplies:

- Amber glass bottles (5ml, 10ml, 30ml)
- Glass roller bottles (for easy application)

- Glass or BPA-free plastic spray bottles (for room and body sprays)
- Ultrasonic diffuser or nebulizer for inhalation benefits
- Beeswax (for making balms and salves)
- Shea butter or cocoa butter (for body butters and creams)
- Aloe vera gel (for soothing skin blends and cooling recipes)
- Witch hazel (natural astringent for facial mists and toners)
- Epsom salts and Himalayan salt (for bath blends)
- Dried herbs for infusion (see seasonal lists below)

Trusted Sources for Ingredients & Supplies:

- **Young Living Essential Oils** (*www.youngliving.com*) – High-quality therapeutic-grade essential oils
- **Mountain Rose Herbs** (*www.mountainroseherbs.com*) – Organic essential oils, carrier oils, dried herbs, beeswax, and DIY supplies
- **Abundant Health™** (*www.abundanthealth4u.com*) – essential oil accessories and blending supplies
- **AromaTools®** (*www.aromatools.com*) – Essential oil bottles, storage, and blending tools recommended for DIY use

PART V
PRACTICAL TIPS & ALCHEMICAL LIVING

In this final section, we bring everything together, exploring practical ways to integrate the wisdom and seasonal insights shared throughout this book.

A significant part of the journey of personal Alchemy and navigating the changing cycles in life, is recognizing the role of grief—not as something to be "fixed" or simply moved past, but as an essential part of our wholeness. Grief is a teacher, a sacred force that allows us to release, grow, and transform.

Just as the cycles of nature remind us that loss and renewal are intertwined, embracing our losses with awareness and compassion enables us to navigate life's transitions with greater resilience and self-understanding.

To support this process, we'll explore ten practical tips to help you integrate these teachings, ensuring that they remain accessible and useful in your daily rhythm.

Additionally, a final reflection offers space for contemplation, inviting you to pause, acknowledge your growth, and step forward with a renewed sense of balance and purpose.

May we remember that just as the darkest night gives way to morning light, grief—when fully acknowledged—has the power to heal, offering not just closure, but a profound opening into a richer, more embodied experience of life.

22
INTEGRATION AND TRANSITION

Honoring the Cycles of Life: Adapting to Change and Embracing Grief

The changing of seasons is more than just a shift in the natural world—it is an invitation for us to align with the rhythms of life. Just as nature transitions from the vibrant energy of spring to the warmth of summer, then to the introspection of autumn, and finally to the stillness of winter, we too are called to embrace these cycles within ourselves. Traditional Chinese Medicine (TCM) and yogic philosophy teach us that adapting to these natural transitions is essential for maintaining balance, resilience, and well-being.

When we learn to flow with nature's rhythms, we cultivate a deeper awareness of ourselves and our connection to the world. This awareness fosters not only harmony but also a sense of non-attachment—allowing us to navigate inevitable changes with grace and openness. By recognizing that change is a natural and necessary part of life, we develop a greater ability to release what no longer serves us and embrace the opportunities for renewal that each season brings.

FINDING BALANCE IN TIMES OF CHANGE

Seasonal shifts are not just external—they are deeply felt within all living beings. Just as trees shed their leaves in autumn or animals enter hibernation in winter, we, too, undergo inner transitions throughout the year. These transitions often bring moments of both growth and loss, reminding us of the impermanence of all things.

Loss, whether the passing of a loved one, the end of a relationship, or the more subtle grief of unfulfilled expectations, is an inherent part of the human experience.

However, in modern society, grief is often overlooked or suppressed. When unexpressed, grief can linger in the body, manifesting as physical ailments, emotional numbness, or a sense of disconnection.

As Sobonfu Somé, a respected West African teacher on grief, reminds us: *"Grief and gratitude are two sides of the same coin. By holding both in our hands, we connect to life in its fullest expression."*

In honoring both grief and gratitude, we acknowledge the depth of our love and the preciousness of life itself.

THE SACRED ROLE OF GRIEF IN OUR LIVES

Many ancient traditions recognized grief as a sacred process, one that required space, ritual, and community support. Today, however, much of this wisdom has been lost, and unexpressed grief has become a silent burden that contributes to emotional and physical distress of our society. I believe this suppression of grief plays a significant role in the dis-ease and disconnection so many experience today.

Grieving is not something to "fix" or rush through—it is something to *honor*. By allowing ourselves to feel and express grief fully, we validate not only the loss but also the love and connection that existed. This process can open us to deeper self-awareness and healing.

As the poet Yehuda HaLevi so beautifully expressed:

"'Tis a fearful thing to love what death can touch...
A holy thing, a holy thing to love."

Grief, then, is not just sorrow—it is a testament to our love, our humanity, and the sacredness of life itself.

GRIEF IN CHINESE MEDICINE: THE IMPACT ON THE BODY AND SPIRIT

In Traditional Chinese Medicine, grief is associated with the Lungs and Heart, which correspond to the Metal and Fire elements, respectively. When grief remains unprocessed, it can create blockages in these energetic systems, leading to physical symptoms such as:

- **Respiratory issues**-asthma, shortness of breath, allergies
- **Tightness in the chest** or difficulty breathing
- **Weakened immunity**-frequent colds, fatigue)
- **Heart-related imbalances**-palpitations, high blood pressure, feelings of heartbreak

Acknowledging and expressing grief is essential for allowing it to move through us rather than becoming stuck in our bodies. Breath work, movement practices, and emotional release techniques can all aid in this process, supporting both physical and emotional well-being.

SUPPORTING GRIEF WITH AROMATHERAPY

Aromatherapy is a powerful tool for emotional healing, as scent has a direct pathway to the brain's limbic system, which governs emotions and memory.

Certain essential oils can help create a soothing, supportive environment for processing grief:

- **Frankincense** – Grounding and centering; promotes inner peace.
- **Lavender** – Calming and restorative; eases anxiety and tension.
- **Rose** – Associated with love and compassion; helps open the heart.
- **Bergamot** – Uplifting and balancing; combats sadness and depression.
- **Neroli** – Comforting and soothing; helps release emotional distress.

These oils can be diffused, added to a warm bath, or applied topically (properly diluted) to encourage relaxation and emotional healing.

HONOR THE INTERCONNECTEDNESS OF MIND, BODY, AND NATURE

True well-being is not just a personal experience—it is deeply connected to the rhythms of nature, our relationships, and the cycles of life. When we nourish our physical health through proper nutrition, movement, and self-care, we create a foundation for vitality. When we tend to our emotional and spiritual health through mindfulness, breath work, and meaningful rituals, we cultivate resilience and inner peace.

Embracing the seasons of life—both joyful and sorrowful—allows us to fully engage with the richness of our existence. By learning to flow with nature's rhythms, we invite a deeper sense of aliveness into our daily lives, honoring every stage of our journey with presence, reverence, love and gratitude.

23
10 KEYS

KEYS TO TRANSFORMATION: UNLOCK YOUR INNER POTENTIAL

Healing is not just about understanding concepts—it's about applying what we've learned in order to create meaningful and lasting change.

Here, we explore a few "Keys" for Alchemical Living, including daily rituals, mindfulness techniques, and simple lifestyle practices to enhance vitality, creativity, and inner balance without costing a lot or taking a ton of effort or time to implement.

These keys can serve as guides for navigating life's transitions with greater ease, helping to foster deeper self-awareness, and cultivate resilience. By embracing these principles, we can align with the ever-evolving nature of existence, allowing transformation to unfold from within.

Below is a summary of my favorite "keys" that can help unlock our true potential. It is not an exhaustive list but covers some very good basics.

May these 10 keys empower you to unlock the doors to a more vibrant, purposeful, and connected life!

1) Practice Supportive Inner Dialogue

- The words you speak to yourself are the most powerful words you can hear. Begin to foster a dialogue of kindness, encouragement, and self-love. Speak to yourself as a compassionate friend, and remember that you are worthy of love, care, healing and second chances.
- Believe in your divine heritage and honor the intrinsic value you hold.
- Ask questions that highlight your gains, instead of focusing on the gaps.
- You are your best source of inner support!

2) Honor the Importance of Rest

- -Rest is essential for your body and mind to replenish. Aim to sleep between 10 pm and 6 am, allowing your body to complete its natural detoxification processes. This aligns with the traditional Chinese medicine cycle, which connects the liver and lungs to Phase 1 and Phase 2 detoxification.
- Sleep during these hours rejuvenates your health on both physical and energetic levels.

3) Incorporate Movement Every Day

- Movement supports the flow of Qi (energy) throughout your body. Whether through yoga asanas, qigong, walking, dancing, or any form that brings joy to your body, make movement a regular part of your day.
- Remember to engage mindfully—lift the crown of your head, lengthen through the spine, and relax the jaw, releasing tension from your neck and shoulders.

- Invite a sense of ease and increasing spaciousness with every movement.

4) Embrace the Wisdom of Your Intuition

- Trust your intuition—listen to your gut feelings and the whispers of your heart. Your body is a powerful source of knowledge, and your intuition holds the key to your well-being! You are literally designed to know what is right for you, but it can take some practice and guidance at first.
- By honoring your inner wisdom, you align with your highest potential and make choices that support your health, happiness, and fulfillment, as well as that of others.

5) Connect with Nature's Healing Presence

- Spend time in nature each day. Set aside at least twenty minutes to sit outside, breathe in fresh air, and reconnect with the natural world. Feel the earth beneath your feet and absorb the tranquility of the natural environment. Nature has a restorative effect on your body and soul, calming the nervous system and promoting balance without any effort.

6) Adapt, Adjust, Accommodate!

- A little yogic rhyme from Swami Sivananda in Rishikiesh that invites us to lean in to a more co-operative attitude with life. Just as the seasons shift, so too can our routines, foods, thoughts, ideas and movements. If we were to travel somewhere for example, we would need to adjust in many different ways to that new environment.
- When you adapt your lifestyle to support your nervous system and immune system during times of transition- you can begin accepting and embracing change with gentleness can help you stay resilient and avoid stagnation in the future.

- Shift your routines intentionally throughout the year to avoid burnout and seasonal imbalances.

7) Find Stability Amidst Change

- While it's important to allow for change, maintaining regularity in certain areas of your life can bring a sense of stability and well-being, and is often another Key to our ultimate sense of satisfaction.
- A balance of both adaptability and stability allows you to adjust to the evolving needs of your body, environment, and lifestyle. What brings you stability today might shift in the future—and that's perfectly okay! Stability doesn't have to mean rigidity but rather a flexible foundation that supports you daily, through life's ebbs and flows.

8) Cultivate Daily Rituals for Health

- Create daily rituals and habits that nurture your physical, emotional, and spiritual well-being. Whether it's a morning meditation, an evening stretch, creating a nature altar for the season, or a nourishing meal, small practices can infuse your day with purpose, intention, and a sense of magic. These rituals help bring you into harmony with yourself and the world around you.

9) Take Regular Tech Breaks

- Technology can be overwhelming to our senses, so it's essential to take intentional breaks from screens. Step away from devices to allow your mind to rest. Stretch your eyes, neck, body and brain, and give yourself space to be present in the moment. This practice fosters mindfulness, enhances productivity, and promotes overall well-being.

10) Embrace your inherent worth and Uniqueness

- When we learn to honor and value both ourselves and others for our unique qualities, we reduce suffering and create space for greater harmony and fulfillment. Your time, energy, ideas, voice, presence, love, and contributions matter —deeply and inherently.
- If you find yourself in an environment where you feel unseen or unappreciated, recognize it as a contrast—a reminder of what it feels like when we are not truly acknowledged, not who you really are!
- Seek out spaces and people who uplift and support your authentic self, where your presence is celebrated and your gifts are valued.
- Honor yourself by nurturing what brings you joy and fulfillment. Surround yourself with those who see and appreciate you for who you truly are. Trust that who you are and what you offer is more than enough.
- And if honoring yourself feels difficult right now, extend yourself the same compassion you would offer a dear friend. Healing and self-worth take time—keep going, keep growing, and continue recognizing all that is beautiful and good within you.

24
A FINAL REFLECTION

As we arrive at the conclusion of this exploration, I invite you to pause and reflect on the journey we have taken together—one that has spanned an entire year perhaps, woven through the ever-changing seasons. Each chapter has opened doors to new perspectives, practices, and insights, offering tools to nourish your body, mind, and spirit in alignment with the rhythms of nature.

Throughout this book, we have explored the wisdom of modern Science, Chinese Medicine, Feng Shui, Yoga, Qigong, Nutrition, Aromatherapy, and more—timeless traditions that remind us of the intricate connection between our physical, emotional, and energetic well-being. As we embrace these connections, we deepen our understanding of ourselves and our place within the greater dance of life.

What have you noticed along the way? Has anything shifted within you? Perhaps a newfound awareness has emerged, or a particular practice has begun to resonate more deeply. This is the beauty of the journey—small shifts, when embraced with intention, create profound transformations over time.

From the vibrant rebirth of spring to the radiant energy of summer, through late summer's harvest, the grounding embrace of autumn, and into the reflective stillness of winter, we have come to understand that each season carries its own lessons and gifts. Just as nature moves through cycles of growth, release, nourishment and rest, so too do we.

Healing is not a singular event but an ever-evolving process—a spiral journey that invites us to listen, honor, and align with both our inner and outer landscapes.

As we close this chapter of our conversation, I hope these teachings and practices continue to serve as gentle reminders on your path. May they inspire you to cultivate curiosity, self-care, compassion, and mindfulness in your daily life. Let gratitude guide you as you honor the sacred interconnectedness of all things.

Above all, remember that *YOU* are the architect of your own wellness. The wisdom, resilience, and healing you seek are already within you, waiting to be nurtured and expressed. Trust in your body's intelligence, your spirit's guidance, and your innate ability to navigate life's challenges with grace and love.

The road ahead may not always be clear, but with the tools you now hold and a steadfast belief in your capacity for transformation, you will find your way. Embrace uncertainty, welcome change, and lean into the unknown with an open heart. With patience and steady practice, you will continue to expand, evolve, and flourish.

May your journey be filled with joy, peace, and the deep knowing that you are a vital and irreplaceable part of this beautiful mystery we call Life. With each step forward, may you walk with intention, reverence, and love—for yourself, for others, and for the world around you.

"I salute the light within your eyes where the whole Universe dwells. For when you are at that center within you and I am at that place within me, we shall be one."

~Namaste~

BIBLIOGRAPHY

CHINESE MEDICINE & TRADITIONAL HEALING SYSTEMS

- Beinfield, Harriet, and Efrem Korngold. *Between Heaven and Earth: A Guide to Chinese Medicine.* Ballantine Books, 1992.
- Jarrett, Lonny S. *Nourishing Destiny: The Inner Tradition of Chinese Medicine.* Spirit Path Press, 1998.
- Maciocia, Giovanni. *The Foundations of Chinese Medicine: A Comprehensive Text for Acupuncturists and Herbalists.* Churchill Livingstone, 2005.
- Ni, Mao Shing. *The Yellow Emperor's Classic of Medicine: A New Translation of the Neijing Suwen with Commentary.* Shambhala Publications, 1995.
- Pitchford, Paul. *Healing with Whole Foods: Asian Traditions and Modern Nutrition.* North Atlantic Books, 2002.
- Huangdi Neijing (The Yellow Emperor's Inner Classic). Han Dynasty (206 BCE – 220 CE).

ONLINE RESOURCES FOR ACUPUNCTURE AND TCM

- National Certification Commission for Acupuncture and Oriental Medicine (NCCAOM) *https://www.nccaom.org/*
- National Center for Complementary and Integrative Health (NCCIH): *https://www.nccih.nih.gov/health/mind-and-body-practices*
- Traditional Chinese Medicine World Foundation: *https://www.tcmworld.org*
- Cleveland Clinic: *https://my.clevelandclinic.org/health/treatments/4767-acupuncture*
- Bastyr University: *https://bastyr.edu/*

SACRED GEOMETRY, FENG SHUI & ENERGY HEALING

- Lieben, John Oscar. *Sacred Geometry for Artists, Dreamers, and Philosophers: Secrets of Harmonic Creation.* Inner Traditions, 2018.
- Becker, Marshall, and Richard Feather Anderson. *The Sacred Geometry Guidebook.* Inner Pathway Publishing, 2016.

BA GUA AND FENG SHUI RESOURCES:

- QC Design School. "Feng Shui Course Sample: Tips for Drawing the Ba Gua Map.": *https://www.qcdesignschool.com/2018/03/feng-shui-course-sample-tips-drawing-the-bagua-map/*
- Young, Stephen Skinner. *The Complete Feng Shui Handbook.* Tuttle Publishing, 1999.
- International Feng Shui Guild: *https://www.ifsguild.org*

YOGA, SOMATIC HEALING & TRAUMA RECOVERY

- Saraswati, Swami Satyananda. *Yoga Nidra.* Bihar School of Yoga, 2009.
- Saraswati, Swami Satyananda. *Asana, Pranayama, Mudra, Bandha.* Bihar School of Yoga, 1969.
- Iyengar, B.K.S. *Light on Yoga.* Schocken Books, 1979.
- Levine, Peter A. *Waking the Tiger: Healing Trauma.* North Atlantic Books, 1997.
- Schwartz, Richard C. *No Bad Parts: Healing Trauma and Restoring Wholeness with the Internal Family Systems Model.* Sounds True, 2021.
- Apigian, Dr. Aimie. *Trauma Healing Accelerated. https://www.traumahealingaccelerated.com*
- The Embody Lab. *Somatic Healing & Trauma Recovery Resources. https://www.embodylab.com*
- Somatic Experiencing International: *https://traumahealing.org*

SOUND HEALING & COLOR THERAPY

- Goldman, Jonathan. *Healing Sounds: The Power of Harmonics.* Inner Traditions, 2002.
- Mitchell, Jonathan. *The Healing Power of Sound: Recovery from Life-Threatening Illness Using Sound, Voice, and Music.* Destiny Books, 2000.
- Birren, Faber. *Color Psychology and Color Therapy: A Factual Study of the Influence of Color on Human Life.* Pickle Partners Publishing, 2015.

ONLINE RESOURCES FOR SOUND AND COLOR HEALING

- The Science of Sound Healing: *https://www.healingsounds.com*
- Color Therapy Healing: *https://www.colourtherapyhealing.com*

AROMATHERAPY & ESSENTIAL OILS

- Perkus, Benjamin. *The Aroma Freedom Technique: Using Essential Oils to Transform Your Emotions and Realize Your Heart's Desires.* CreateSpace, 2016.
- Tisserand, Robert, and Rodney Young. *Essential Oil Safety: A Guide for Health Care Professionals.* Churchill Livingstone, 2014.
- Young Living Essential Oils: *https://www.youngliving.com*
- Essential Oil Safety Guide: *https://www.youngliving.com/en_US/discover/essential-oil-safety*
- Mountain Rose Herbs: *https://www.mountainroseherbs.com*
- DIY Aromatherapy Resources: *https://www.aromaweb.com*
- Life Science Publishing *www.lifesciencepublishers.com* – Essential oil reference books, roller bottles, diffusers, and storage cases
- Abundant Health® *www.abundanthealth4u.com* – essential oil accessories and blending supplies
- AromaTools® *www.aromatools.com* – Essential oil bottles, storage, and blending tools recommended for DIY use
- National Association for Holistic Aromatherapy: *https://www.naha.org*

HEALTH, ADAPTOGENS, AND THE DEFAULT MODE NETWORK

- Winston, David. *Adaptogens: Herbs for Strength, Stamina, and Stress Relief.* Healing Arts Press, 2007.
- *Default Mode Network & Brain Health Research with PTSD:* National Institutes of Health (NIH): *https://pmc.ncbi.nlm.nih.gov/articles/PMC9986502/*

PINEAL GLAND, CHRISTA GALLI, AND THE THIRD EYE CONNECTION

- Strassman, Rick. *DMT: The Spirit Molecule: A Doctor's Revolutionary Research into the Biology of Near-Death and Mystical Experiences.* Park Street Press, 2001.
- Netter, Frank H. *Atlas of Human Anatomy.* Elsevier, 2018.
- *The Pineal Gland, Aging, Melatonin & Sleep Regulation https://pmc.ncbi.nlm.nih.gov/articles/PMC6017004/*

REIKI & ENERGY HEALING

- Rand, William Lee. *The Healing Touch: The Definitive Guide to Reiki Practice.* Sounds True, 2016.

- Takata, Hawayo. *Reiki: Hawayo Takata's Story*. Lotus Light Publications, 2003.
- International Center for Reiki Training: *https://www.reiki.org*

GENERAL WELLNESS & MINDFULNESS

- Hanh, Thich Nhat. *Peace Is Every Step: The Path of Mindfulness in Everyday Life*. Bantam Books, 1991.
- A Positive Mindset Can Help Your Heart: *https://www.health.harvard.edu/blog/a-positive-mindset-can-help-your-heart-2019021415999*
- The Importance of Sleep for Immune Health: *https://www.nhlbi.nih.gov/health-topics/education-and-awareness/sleep-health*

AFTERWORD

THE INSPIRATION BEHIND THE ALCHEMY OF WELLNESS

The book was born from a deep-seated curiosity, love of healing, and lifelong fascination with alchemy—not just as a mystical process, but as a way of blending the practical with the spiritual, the ancient with the modern, and the personal with the universal.

It reflects my heartfelt desire to bridge these worlds, offering an accessible guide for transformation and well-being to all who walk the path.

It is a culmination of my own lived experiences, decades of study and practice, and the profound insights gained from working with thousands of patients and students as an acupuncturist, yoga teacher, and Reiki energy healer over these last twenty years. The seeds of this book were planted during my early studies of Chinese medicine in China and my immersion in Yoga philosophy in ashrams in India.

I became fascinated by how seamlessly these ancient systems of healing intertwined with the cycles of nature, the rhythms of the seasons, and the sensory experiences that make us human.

Over time, my exploration deepened to naturally include other forms of body work, aromatherapy, nutrition, poetry, and complementary modalities, all of which enriched the access to healing and a felt sense of wholeness for myself, clients and students.

The true spark for compiling this book has always been from my patients and students. Over the years, I was asked time and again to write, teach, video or share more of what I was offering in sessions and classes. I was busy seeing patients and teaching and did not find the time to create those things... Until now!

Over the years, I have witnessed firsthand how reconnecting with the body, senses, and natural world significantly enhances our well-being. It is not a matter of belief, but of following age old natural principles. Whether through breath work, Acupuncture, Reiki, mindful movement, time in nature, or the healing power of essential oils, we each can rediscover a sense of wholeness and vitality that we may not have even known was missing.

This alchemy of re connection and transformation inspired me to create a guide that is simple, practical, and accessible—no matter where you are on your journey or how familiar you are with ancient wisdom and practices.

As I wrote The Alchemy of Wellness, I reflected often on my own path and all I have learned along the way.

While attending Bastyr University-a Naturopathic Medical school in Kenmore, WA, I sought out many teachers and healing modalities and immersed myself fully in experiencing and learning from all of them. I was honestly obsessed with learning everything I could and experiencing new ways to help myself and others.

A medical intuitive once told me at a Women of Wisdom conference in Seattle in my early twenties that-" I would be a "bridge between East and West"—a statement I did not really understand at the time, but a role that has proven to be true over and over again as I reflect back.

By teaching and reminding others of these ancient, powerful practices and perspectives, I have fulfilled this bridging destiny in many ways over the past two decades.

Like so many, of course I have faced challenges, doubts, and times of deep transformation along the way—my own Hero's Journey if you will.

Through it all, I have come to understand the importance of honoring and nurturing all aspects of being—mind, body, and spirit—and the power of aligning with life's natural rhythms and cycles, especially during challenging times.

My intention is for this book to be more than just a collection of tools and techniques. It is an invitation—to reconnect with yourself, with nature, and with the bigger picture rhythms that sustain us all.

I hope it has inspired you to slow down, notice, savor and embrace the beauty of life in all its "seasons".

LOOKING AHEAD

If *The Alchemy of Wellness* has resonated with you, I invite you to continue this journey with me. I am dedicated to sharing wisdom, guidance, and practices through workshops, retreats, and online platforms.

Currently, I am working on several new projects, including:

- An audio version of this book! Available soon on audible.com
- Guided audio journeys to support your seasonal explorations
- Future offerings and classes designed to enhance your well-being
- A new APP with all the how to's and audio/video guidance for the practices.

You can find updates, additional resources, and information about my offerings by visiting *www.quantumpurposecoach.com* or connecting with me on social media.

SUPPORT OUR GRASSROOTS MISSION – LEAVE AN AMAZON REVIEW

I sincerely hope this book has provided you with inspiration, insight, and practical tools to integrate ancient wisdom into your present day life.

If this book has resonated with you in any way, one of the most impactful ways you can support this work is by leaving an honest review on Amazon. Your review is more than just a few words—it's a powerful way to help others discover this book and embark on their own healing journey.

Why Your Review Matters

This project is a grassroots effort, created with the intention of bringing holistic healing and seasonal wisdom to as many people as possible. Unlike large publishing houses with massive marketing budgets, independent books like this thrive on word-of-mouth recommendations and personal connections. Your review plays a vital role in:

Helping Others Find the Book – Amazon's search algorithms prioritize books with more reviews, making it easier for those who need this wisdom to find it.

Building a Community – Your words may inspire someone else to start their own healing journey, creating a ripple effect of wellness and transformation.

Supporting Independent Authors – By taking a few moments to leave a review, you help amplify this work and sustain the creation of more content that blends ancient traditions with modern healing.

How to Leave a Review

Leaving a review is simple and takes just a few minutes:

- **Go to the Amazon page** where you purchased *The Alchemy of Wellness*.
- **Scroll down** to the "Customer Reviews" section.
- **Click "Write a Review"** and rate the book using the star system.
- **Share your thoughts**—What did you enjoy most? Did any practices or insights resonate with you? How has this book influenced your wellness journey?
- **Click "Submit"**—and that's it!

What to Write?

Your review doesn't have to be long—just a few sentences about what you found valuable or meaningful is incredibly helpful. Consider mentioning:

- How the book has helped you in your personal wellness journey
- Your favorite section or practice
- Why you would recommend it to others
- Any positive changes you've noticed since applying the insights in the book

From the bottom of my heart, thank you for being part of this grassroots movement to bring deeper awareness and connection to the world. Your support allows this work to grow, reach more people, and continue evolving into future offerings.

I am deeply grateful for your time, energy, and presence on this journey. Thank you for leaving a review and for helping share *The Alchemy of Wellness* with those who are seeking a path to greater balance, health, and inner harmony!

ABOUT THE AUTHOR

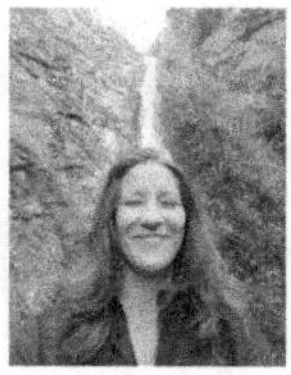

Erika holds a Masters Degree from Bastyr University in Kenmore, WA. She graduated in 2005 with a specialty in Acupuncture and Chinese Medicine.

Her studies and specialties during her career have included Acupuncture, Cupping, Herbology, Nutrition, Yoga, Qigong, Tai Chi, Reflexology, Holy Fire Reiki, Somatics, Functional Medicine, Aromatherapy, Sound Healing and more.

She retired from hands-on practice in 2022 and is currently focused on offering distance healing, consulting, teaching, writing and utilizing the power of the Human Design system and Quantum principles to help people thrive and learn how to utilize their own energy and personal strategy for healing.

She resides in northern Idaho with her husband, Gere, and their sweet dog, Ruby. Her favorite source of joy and alignment is spending time in nature with them throughout the beautiful seasons; hiking, biking, nordic skiing and canoeing!

https://www.quantumpurposecoach.com/thealchemyofwellness

www.ingramcontent.com/pod-product-compliance
Lightning Source LLC
LaVergne TN
LVHW052300200926
848481LV00002B/419
* 9 7 9 8 3 4 9 2 1 4 4 3 1 *